Born to Walk

Myofascial Efficiency and the Body in Movement

James Earls

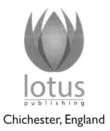

lotus
publishing

Chichester, England

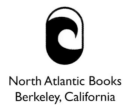

North Atlantic Books
Berkeley, California

First published in 2014 by
Lotus Publishing
Apple Tree Cottage, Inlands Road, Nutbourne, Chichester, PO18 8RJ and
North Atlantic Books
P.O. Box 12327
Berkeley, California 94712

Drawings Amanda Williams
Text Design Wendy Craig
Cover Design Paula Morrison
Printed and Bound in Malaysia by Tien Wah Press

Born to Walk: Myofascial Efficiency and the Body in Movement is sponsored by the Society for the Study of Native Arts and Sciences, a nonprofit educational corporation whose goals are to develop an educational and cross-cultural perspective linking various scientific, social, and artistic fields; to nurture a holistic view of arts, sciences, humanities, and healing; and to publish and distribute literature on the relationship of mind, body, and nature.

British Library Cataloguing-in-Publication Data
A CIP record for this book is available from the British Library
ISBN 978 1 905367 47 4 (Lotus Publishing)
ISBN 978 1 58394 769 2 (North Atlantic Books)

Library of Congress Cataloguing-in-Publication Data
Earls, James, author.
  Born to walk : myofascial efficiency and the body in movement / James Earls.
    p. ; cm.
  ISBN 978-1-58394-769-2
  I. Title.
  [DNLM: 1. Walking—physiology. 2. Biomechanical Phenomena. 3. Gait—physiology. 4. Musculoskeletal Physiological Phenomena. WE 103]
  RA781.65
  613.7'176—dc23
                              2014007920

Contents

Foreword

It is a great pleasure to introduce readers to incisive ideas. James Earls is a critical thinker; when he applies his brain to a question like gait, the result is worth the effort to read and understand. This is true of *Born to Walk,* where human plantigrade posture and bipedal gait are given the full circle of his imaginative but no-nonsense treatment.

It is also a great personal pleasure, of course, to see the ideas of *Anatomy Trains,* first published in 1997, taken up and expanded into this bold new work. The application of the Anatomy Trains myofascial meridian lines in the dynamics of gait (rather than the compensatory patterns of posture, as it was originally put into practice) is an exciting new direction for the Anatomy Trains model.

We live in a dynamic era, poised atop two crucial turning points. One is the dynamic between the "old" anatomy—the reductive anatomy of the musculoskeletal system as we have understood it since Vesalius—and the more "holistic" vision implied by the Anatomy Trains model, fractal mathematics, systems theory, and a host of recent research on myofascial force transmission. The attempt in *Anatomy Trains,* and certainly the attempt here in this book, is to bend these two ends and make them meet.

"Particulate" anatomy—"this muscle goes from origin to insertion and thus performs this set of actions"—is clearly inadequate to explain what is going on during daily coordinated movement. On the other hand, the holistic premise—"everything is connected to everything else"—while true, leaves the questioner in a vacuous world where everything is possible. So how do we strategize? How do we decide where to go and what to do next and when we are finished?

The "parts" view and the holistic view must be married, and *Born to Walk* gets them at least affianced, if not all the way down the aisle. The physiotherapist will find much in this book to get his or her teeth into in terms of specifics and isolating tests for determining the site of malfunction, and the model is built on classic gait theory. The holistic practitioner will likewise find much to fill in the "everything's connected" trope with practical advice as to how to see, assess, and work with the whole person in motion.

The second turning point we are at, in this early part of the twenty-first century, is the increasing amount of somatic alienation and "sensori-motor amnesia" that we see in our texting young, our sedentary workers, and our debilitated elderly. Clearly, we need an integrated approach to "KQ" (Kinesthetic Intelligence, Movement Literacy) for our urbanized populace—a group that includes more than just city dwellers. I live in a town of six hundred souls in a lovely, rural part of the United States, but I still live an entirely "urbanized" life.

Aside from educating current and upcoming generations, we need to educate our professional brethren. The emerging field of "Spatial Medicine"—changing the body position or movement to change the person—will bring together orthopedic doctors, physiatrists, physiotherapists, osteopaths, chiropractors, personal trainers, Pilates and yoga teachers, bodyworkers and manual therapists of all stripes, and somatic educators like Alexander Technique teachers and Feldenkrais practitioners. In my experience, each of us has something to learn from all these approaches, each of which have something to offer the whole field, and each separate school of thought has much to learn from the other parts of the field.

Over the next generation, all these tender "shoots" will eventually bind into a strong and comprehensive theory of anthropological development, biomechanics, physical education, rehabilitation, and skill maintenance that will promote a functional body, no matter what one's individual circumstances are. As we move behind the tail of the Industrial Revolution and enter the mouth of the Electronic Era, this effort—to reach out, understand the value in other approaches, and to apply the results toward a grand theory—will take on greater and greater significance, as our children's connection with nature is curtailed and "virtual reality" becomes less virtual and more palpably real.

Born to Walk is a vital step along this path, the bringing together of the holistic and the classical view to understand the uniqueness of human gait in terms that are both practical and visionary, scientific and poetic, grounded and uplifting.

I enjoy the book you have in your hands, and I expect that you will too.

Thomas Myers
Clarks Cove, Maine
November 11, 2013

Introduction

Man is a model of the world.
—Leonardo da Vinci c. 1480

"Vitruvian Man," Leonardo da Vinci's instantly recognizable sketch of the proportions of man, is a powerful symbol that demonstrates the relationship between architecture and anatomy and has been a source of inspiration for artists and architects over the centuries (fig. 0.1). Yet it is also one of the clearest expressions of the reasons for our limitations in the study of anatomy over the last 3,700 years.

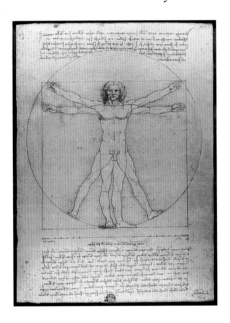

Figure 0.1. "Vitruvian Man" by Leonardo da Vinci, c. 1487.
Along with the accompanying text, it outlines the ideal human proportions and is sometimes referred to as the "Canon of Proportions" or "Proportions of Man."

We can't really blame Leonardo, however. The symbol was drawn at a time of human history when we knew no better. In fact, the sketch was probably the epitome of the contemporary thinking of the Renaissance. Da Vinci made concrete and visible the ideal relationships between human anatomy, the divine, and the universe, as described by Vitruvius.

Writing sometime around 20 BCE, Vitruvius was instructed by the emperor Augustus to redesign, reformulate, and reinvigorate the beleaguered Roman Empire. Vitruvius wanted to establish a new format for the design of towns and buildings, and Augustus wanted a "Corpus," literally a body of work that would encapsulate the reformation of the "body of the empire." Vitruvius's *De architectura libri decum* (Ten books on architecture) was the outcome. It was the first work to outline the role and aspiration of an architect, and it sought to define many of the necessary elements of architecture.

Vitruvius's fundamental tenet was that "the power of nature has acted as architect" in biology: universal laws of nature had brought about human anatomy, and so, within our body's design, we had a map of the macrocosm. The body was literally a *minor mundus*, a "mini world," and, thereby, a reflection of the universe. The implication was that the architect should apply the wisdom and proportions of the body's design to architectural design and creation: "No temple can be put together coherently without symmetry and proportions unless it conforms exactly to the principle relating to the members of a well-shaped man."

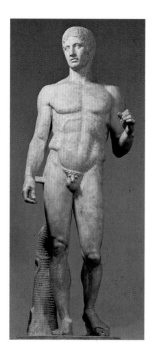

Figure 0.2. The statue of the spear-bearer by the Greek sculptor Polykleitos was originally created 450–400 BCE. It was referenced by many as an example of the ideal proportions of a man, including Galen, the hugely influential physician, six hundred years later, as well as by Vitruvius and, eventually, by da Vinci.

In drawing Vitruvian Man, da Vinci wanted to demonstrate his mastery of anatomy and his understanding of the divine, as well as his mechanical and architectural prowess. By encapsulating the human form within the circle and the square, he was demonstrating the divine and the earthly relationships of the body, the slight upward shift of the circle allowing the navel to become the geometric center as well as a physiological one. The problem is that he operated with the tools of the time: a set square and a compass. In doing so, Leonardo set a foundation stone of anatomical misunderstanding within the modern world, by setting out a geometrical perfection of anatomy that would be associated with the tools and methods of fifteenth-century construction.

The use of the human body as the model for architecture lasted for many centuries. The body was used to inspire architecture, and the inverse was applied as well, with architecture and the idea of bricks and mortar being used to build an understanding of anatomy. Herein lies the problem with our traditional analysis of anatomy.

We naturally understand the progression of setting one brick on top of another—most of us have been doing that experiment since we first sat up and began playing with blocks. It is one of our first learned constants of the world: the relationship between gravity, inertia, and balance. Just as we used the body to inform architecture, over the centuries we have used our understanding of architecture to inform our experiments with the body. We have walked a two-way street with one discipline informing the other.

Many anatomy books still use the block-type image to portray the human form. It is still a popular depiction within my own profession, structural integration, employed by its originator, Dr. Ida Rolf. The language of engineering has entered the anatomical lexicon with the use of levers, cantilevers, force couples, supports, and attachments. And so we are naturally seduced into seeing anatomy with the same eye that we use to look at the manmade world around us.

While da Vinci may have been the source of this misinformed view of the body, he was also the inspiration for a new way of thinking about the body. Late fifteenth-century thinking was dominated by the Bible and by Aristotelian teachings of the natural and religious worlds. The writings of Galen were almost universally accepted without question. Da Vinci was among the first to start breaking this tradition, separating dogma from observable, demonstrable fact. By separating these two elements within Vitruvian Man—the circle (the divine) and the square (the earthly)—he was anticipating the changes that would develop through the world in the following few centuries.

Immersing himself in anatomy and, in the process, revolutionizing its portrayal, da Vinci began to see that many anatomical features were not as had been described by Galen 1,200 years previously. Many of these mistakes were still being taught in universities and, rather than trust the "wisdom" of his contemporary anatomists, da Vinci undertook many of his own dissections, the sketches of which are now kept as part of the Royal Collection in London.

Da Vinci inspired many scientists to follow in his footsteps. The Belgian anatomist Vesalius (1514–64) took further liberties in challenging the Galenic tradition, and in his dissections at the University of Padua acted as both dissector and lecturer *(ostensor cum sector)*. This went against the established practice of having a dissector *(sector)*, demonstrator *(ostensor)*, and a lecturer *(lector)*. The latter's job was primarily to simply regurgitate the writings of Galen as the dissector cut and the demonstrator pointed to the relevant parts, whether or not they matched the descriptions being given.

Shortly after Vesalius's time in Padua, the English physician William Harvey (1578–1657) also wished to branch out, preferring to believe his observation rather than received wisdom. His persistence—some might say obstinance—resulted in the medical breakthrough of the understanding of the circulation of blood.

Thus scientists in the sixteenth and seventeenth centuries began to challenge the orthodoxy, casting a new light of inspection onto many of the ancient scripts that had hitherto been accepted without question. Everything was up for scrutiny, and thinkers like René Descartes and Francis Bacon gave the world the tools it needed for critical analysis, leading us into the Age of Enlightenment (from around 1650).

The explosion in scientific undertakings in the mid- and late seventeenth century included Huygens (mathematics and astronomy), Boyle (chemistry), Wren (architecture and physics), Leibniz (mathematics), Hevelius (astronomy), Leeuwenhoek (microscopy), and two of our heroes for this book—Isaac Newton (1642–1727) and Robert Hooke (1635–1703).

Newton's work on gravity and motion is familiar to many of us, but the work of Robert Hooke, Newton's contemporary, is less so, even though it covered many more areas and foresaw much that could not be fully understood at that time. To appreciate the benefits of our bipedal gait and our design as nature intended, we must pay homage to the work of both men. We must understand Newton's principles of motion and our interactions with gravity and the ground, but they fully make sense only if we also invoke the elastics of Hooke.

Despite publishing one of the earliest—if not the earliest—close-up images of a flea (fig. 0.3), Robert Hooke only worked with nonorganic elastics and springs, and so we cannot be fully informed by his work. But we will see that the interaction between the principles of gravity and elasticity established by these two men, who at times were adversaries, gives a new understanding on how our bodies function. Hooke has been honored by having the symbol representing the elastic sections in the body named after him (see chapter 1).

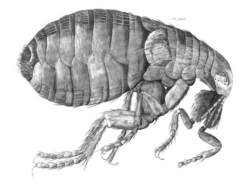

Figure 0.3. Published in 1665, this image, from Micrographica by Robert Hooke, helped to popularize science. It was perhaps the first "popular science" title and included many other firsts, such as the use of the word cell, as well as early work on fossils, predating Darwin by some two hundred years.

It is through the combination of gravity and our tissue's response to our momentum that we can gain practically free energy. By using the body's movement to stretch elastic tissues, we recruit the captured energy and then recoil the kinetic energy (the energy of motion) to help create a return movement. It is to this mechanism that much of this book is dedicated; it gives us the gift of relaxed and graceful movement that we recognize through its ease and the flow through and incorporation of the whole body.

Up until the twentieth century, scientists took a predominately Cartesian approach to the body, concentrating on "parts" and maintaining the image of the body working

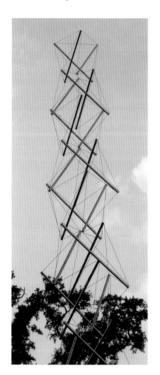

as an architectural machine. This concept of the body was not really challenged until 1948, when the sculptor Kenneth Snelson produced a series of structures that unintentionally imitated the interaction between the bones and the myofascia of the body (see fig. 0.4). Snelson, then studying with the philosopher and architect Buckminster Fuller, used tensioned wires to support solid, compressional struts. Fuller went on to develop the ideas and geometry of what he came to term "tensegrity" structures, using them as models for elements of the natural world from the atom to humanity to the universe (an interesting echo of the earlier natural philosophers' desire to show the geometry of the microcosm matching the macrocosm).

Figure 0.4. Using tensioned wire and metal struts, self-supporting structures can be created. The integrity of the structure requires the interplay between the compression and tension elements. As Snelson points out, however, while the breaking of one element in a simple structure can lead to its collapse, challenging one area in more complex constructions will be less catastrophic (for more, see his website, http://kennethsnelson.net/faq). We will see this again as we look further at the body and how it can adapt to dysfunction in any area.

In Snelson's and Fuller's world, to understand the system, we have to fully comprehend the connecting elements. That universal connecting ingredient in our bodies is the fascial tissue, a previously under appreciated element of our makeup, yet a wondrous multifaceted material that both binds and separates organs, and stabilizes and facilitates the mobility within us.

Now, in the twenty-first century, the fascial system seems to be attracting the attention it deserves. This has been due to the groundwork established by many pioneers, including Ida Rolf (1896–1979) and her many students, Thomas Myers in particular, with his development of the comprehensive fascial map, Anatomy Trains. By combining the principles of the physics of Newton and Hooke; the systems of Fuller and Snelson; the anatomy of Thomas Myers; and the functional movement of other pioneers, such as Jacquelin Perry, Gary Gray, and David Tiberio, I hope that this text can bring a united understanding of one of humanity's defining characteristics, bipedal gait.

This book aims to show that the body is "designed" along the lines of a different model from that extrapolated from the world of masons so beautifully encapsulated by da Vinci in his Vitruvian Man. I hope to show a model that will prove to be far more informative and satisfying, one that allows the whole body to adapt and cooperate with the movement of walking, and one that shows how we utilize the energy-saving mechanisms inherent within our anatomy. And, if I can borrow the words from Newton's reply to Hooke's accusation of plagiarism, if there is anything worthwhile in this book, "if I have seen any further," then it is not through my own efforts, but simply because I have had the opportunity to "stand on the shoulders of ye Giants."

And so I must thank all of those who have given of their time to me: Trefor Campbell, without whom this journey would not have gotten started on this path; Don Thompson and Kathy Green, without whom the journey would be less fun and certainly much longer; Thomas Myers, Art Riggs, and David Tiberio, who made the path smoother and less winding through their guidance; my loving partner, Liza Cawthorn, without whom the journey would have been long and lonely, her kind supportive guidance and affection made this trek smoother and I would certainly not have reached the end without it (plus a huge thanks from every reader for the many hours of editing, the book would not have made sense without it!); and, of course, my parents, without both of them the first steps would never have been taken. Thanks to my long suffering support team at Lotus Publishing, Simon Chiu for his expert technical support, Amanda for her patience as I often read the map upside down or back to front and we had to double back a few times, Wendy for her clarity in putting the map on the page, and, of course Jon who let us go on this saunter together.

Solvitur ambulando, St. Jerome was fond of saying. To solve a problem, walk around.
—Gregory McNamee

People usually consider walking on water or in thin air a miracle. But I think the real miracle is not to walk either on water or in thin air, but to walk on earth. Every day we are engaged in a miracle which we don't even recognize: a blue sky, white clouds, green leaves, the black, curious eyes of a child—our own two eyes. All is a miracle.
—Thich Nhat Hanh

The "Walking System"

The body divides itself into two units: passenger and locomotor.... The passenger unit is responsible only for its own postural integrity.
—Jacquelin Perry, *Gait Analysis*

But

Walking while nursing an injured arm in a cast throws off your balance and distorts your geometry of the walking body, creating various tensions and asymmetries that in themselves create further pain. My broken arm ached and it made the rest of my body ache, too.
—**Geoffrey Nicholson**, *The Lost Art of Walking*

Walking on two legs requires a tremendous act of balance and is often described as "controlled falling"—if we do not successfully put one foot in front of the other, we'll fall to the ground. For our four-legged friends, walking must be so much easier, as they always have at least two points of contact with the ground at any one time. For us, walking requires the ability to have just one foot on the ground and to maintain some form of equilibrium within our tall, straight, and very unstable structures.

We walk to move around, to take our head and hands to other places, to achieve needs and desires. This apparently simple action requires a brain and nervous system; it demands internal planning and an ability to predict actions and reactions. It makes use of the many other cooperative senses that we have developed over millions of years. For elegant and efficient walking, each of our "systems"—especially those of sight, balance, and sensation—must be communicating in harmony. This requires the coordination abilities of the brain and nervous system.

One of the inherent problems in the study of anatomy is that we organize anatomy by these "systems." In breaking the organization of the body down into similar tissue types, we tend to focus our attention on just one system at a time. Ideally, we should talk about the "walking system" throughout this book, but, alas, that would be a much larger tome, and it would require knowledge beyond my capabilities. Therefore, I must limit myself to analyzing the body's neuro-myo-fascial-skeletal-vestibular system, and my main focus will be on the myofascial elements and their cooperation.

Homo sapiens developed as generalists; we can adapt to many different situations, weaknesses, and disabilities. A glance at the people on any city street will quickly demonstrate various strategies for what we call "walking." There are many factors—neurological, visceral, emotional, cultural, and structural—that can alter how we walk. The number of possible interactions within those factors would be too large to list and would possibly require consultation with just as many professionals to unravel. It is for that reason that I will concentrate on developing a model of "normal," nonpathological gait.

This book presents a version of what can happen when the whole body is allowed to move together. I hesitate to call it "normal," but it is a pattern that is inherent within most of us—within the lines and grooves, contours and forms of our inherited anatomy. It is the relaxed, repetitive walking that allows our brains to be otherwise occupied, facilitating our gift to "walk and talk," to philosophize, to compose, to fall in love, to meander through any number of human preoccupations. It is a gift eulogized by many—from the peripatetic philosophers to Wordsworth and Dickens—and a facility brought about through what Bernstein (the founder of motor-control theory) referred to as "level B functioning." Walking, according to Bernstein, uses synergy among many different muscles, coordinated without any input from the brain, relying on self-monitoring by the proprioceptive system (Latash 2012). In our exploration of the myofascial system, we will see how the mechanoreceptors are located within the fascial tissue and seem to form a computation system that allows walking to be a subconscious activity.

Your body is built for walking.
—Gary Yanker

I believe the whole body walks. That might sound like a ridiculously obvious thing to say, but many schools of thought exist in the modeling of gait that narrow their gaze to analyzing just one aspect of human motion. One of the most widely accepted theories splits the body into "locomotor" and "passenger" sections—the pelvis and lower limbs versus the head, arms, and trunk (Perry and Burnfield 2010). Another school of thought, put forward by Gracovetsky, suggests that we only require the deep spinal muscles to move (2008). The alternate contraction of the multifidi, he argues, gives us the rotational movement we need to propel ourselves in any direction.

While there is certainly a truth in each of these theories, they are—for me—quite incomplete. We use the whole body to walk: the pelvis and legs are assisted by the trunk and the arms. The whole body helps balance and movement by increasing and decreasing the forces moving through the soft tissue. The whole body also works to lessen the amount of distortion that reaches the head. We need to keep our eyes relatively level, and we certainly do not want the force of impact rattling our brains at each heel strike, so we require the trunk and shoulder girdles to constantly adapt to keep the head steady.

The three elements of the walking system I will focus on most will be the fascial, muscular, and skeletal elements. These combine to form a wonderful, symbiotic map of the forces that travel through the body. The shapes and contours of the bones and their joints create pathways, like dry riverbeds, which, come the flood, will direct the water along preferred paths. The bones and joints assist the body through a controlled pattern of shock absorption, with the folding of joints taking place along predictable lines that send the force of impact into the semifluid streams of myofascial tissue.

The first port of call for our journey through the walking body will be the sequence of events in the bones and joints, in chapter 2. Understanding the natural inclination of the bones and the way they move on impact will allow us to interpret the role of the soft tissues, which—provided the other systems are properly in place—react to the forces by keeping us upright and still moving forward.

The myofascial tissues are not always consciously directed (as most anatomy books say they are) but are often reactive in behavior. For example, the tibialis anterior can be actively contracted to create dorsiflexion and inversion, but its role in walking is to react to the body's interaction with the ground to prevent, control, or slow down plantarflexion and eversion. Its contraction in walking is a response to the lengthening of tissues around it as the foot is planted on the ground—it's a totally unconscious reaction (see fig. 1.1). This reaction is controlled by the proprioceptors in the fascia, and thereby we see the role of the nervous system in this already increasingly complicated story.

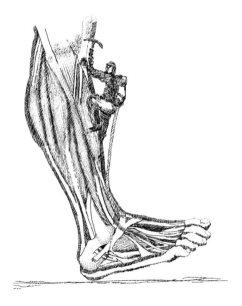

Figure 1.1. The impact of the foot on the ground will send forces into the soft tissue along the channels determined by the joints. These changes are felt by the proprioceptors, and an automatic response is created by the neuromuscular system to control the movement. Through the gait cycle, the tibialis anterior (and all of the other muscle units) will be constantly adjusting its tension in response to the surrounding events, reacting first to the eversion of the calcaneus and then to the ankle plantarflexion (see chapter 3, "Superficial Front and Superficial Back Lines", for further breakdown).

In the morning a man walks with his whole body; in the evening, only with his legs.
—Ralph Waldo Emerson

The body's many proprioceptors are constantly sensing changes in tension and relative position and communicating this information to the appropriate muscles. The wonderful work of Huijing has shown us that the mechanical force at a tendon is not communicated only along the muscle itself but is also dispersed into the surrounding fascia and can therefore be felt by the proprioceptors embedded within neighboring muscles (1999a and 1999b, see fig. 1.2). In this way, a change at one end of a muscle can lead to its many neighbors being stimulated, depending on the pattern of movement.

This means that the fascial tissue of tibialis anterior, for example, can perceive mechanical information not only from its neighbors—extensors hallucis and digitorum longus, fibularis longus and brevis—but also from tibialis posterior or any of the other muscles of the leg. It is constantly receiving three-dimensional information of what is happening in the tissue around it and responding to those changes, creating a four-dimensional assessment and reaction to mechanical forces (time being the fourth dimension). The role of the proprioceptors is covered more fully in chapter 6.

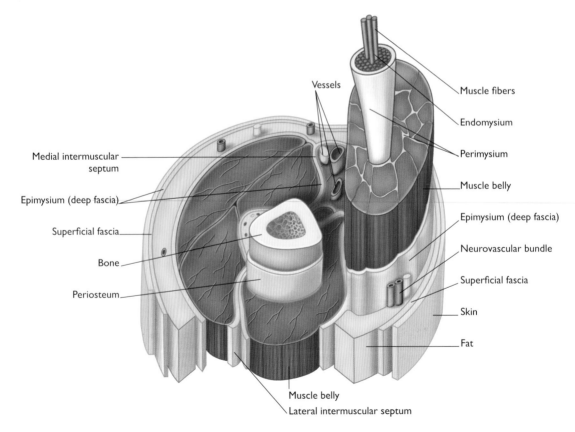

Figure 1.2. Pull or lengthen the distal attachment of any muscle, and that force will go out into the surrounding fascia to be sensed by the proprioceptors. Other myofascial elements can then make appropriate responses to the force in keeping with whatever mechanical information they are receiving from their own four-dimensional environment.

It is that extra dimension of time that makes description of walking so complex, as we have to visualize and analyze our adaptations in the three planes (sagittal, frontal, and transverse) as the body moves through time, changing positions. I hope the analysis put forward in this book helps ease some of that burden.

OUR RELATIONSHIP WITH GRAVITY

Walking is posture in motion.
—Mary Bond, "The New Rules of Posture"

During my training in structural integration, I would often hear the saying (almost a mantra for some people) that we have to live and align ourselves with gravity, that gravity is both our friend and our enemy. This always made perfect sense to me in terms of static postural assessment, in which we can see the impact of imbalanced segments and the strains that gravity causes.

I believe the statement fully comes to life, however, when we see the body working as the "walking system" of the bones, joint alignment, and the neuromyofascial continuum. Our eyes are naturally drawn to efficient, flowing, graceful movement: the joints moving freely in their designated ranges and directions; the myofascia receiving the appropriate information, both from the somatic nervous system and from sensing the mechanics of the surrounding tissue. When all of these happen together, we perceive a harmonious relationship, both of the body within itself and of the body with gravity.

It looks easy because it is. Nothing in the body is being taken advantage of; there is no overextension; and there is movement everywhere. The whole body is working as one to achieve its goal. When this happens, we achieve efficient movement. And strangely, it is the inherent instability of our two-legged stance that produces this efficiency.

UNDERGROUND FORCES AT WORK

"Ground Reaction Force" may sound like a subterranean terrorist group, but it is actually a vitally important aspect of understanding what is happening during gait. Unfortunately, it is also probably one of the most confused aspects. This is the stage where many readers may be tempted to skip a few pages, as they feel the imminence of the "science bit"—but please hold true just for a few pages. It will serve you very well, not just for the rest of this book, but also in the understanding of any human movement.

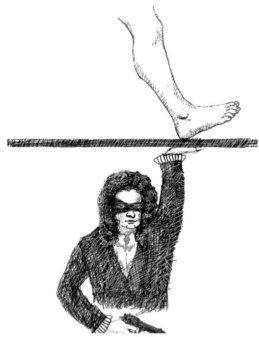

Figure 1.3. Ground reaction force is more complex than a simple rebounding of energy, as would be predicted from a simple understanding of Newton's third law.

One of the problems with explaining ground reaction force is that it begins to invoke physics, and everyone loves to quote Newton's third law: "To every action there is an equal and opposite reaction." What this means is that when my foot hits the ground, the ground pushes right back at me with the same force, but in the opposite direction, and this helps keep me upright. Sometimes in movement classes, instructors encourage their students, "push into the ground and feel it push you back up." Unfortunately, this is a bit of an oversimplification.

Let us begin with the difference between walking on asphalt and walking on sand—we all know the extra work that is needed when sauntering across a beach. Taking the example of the asphalt first: when we push into it, the surface will deform slightly (not enough for us to notice it with ordinary human senses, but it does happen), and it will return to its original state as we push off from it.

When we walk on the beach, however, the force with which we push into the surface is used to displace the many thousands of grains of sand. The grains are not connected to one another, and so the beach does not have an elastic capability to regain its original form. When we heel strike in sand, most of the force is therefore dispersed and gets lost in the movement of the grains.

If we looked very closely at the sand, we could see that the movement of each grain will depend on its shape and the angle from which it is pushed. Because the grains of sand aren't bonded together, these changes are similar to hitting balls on a pool table. Once the force stops acting on the grains (or balls), they come to rest where they are, rather than return to their starting position.

Much of the energy inherent in the foot strike was used up by the displacement of the sand. Now imagine that the grains of sand were joined to one another by strong elastic bands. Each of those movements by the sand would be reversible, just like a trampoline, which is temporarily displaced but, due to its elasticity, returns to its original shape— and thereby returns the energy used to displace it by pushing the person who jumped on it into the air.

Until now we have considered the body as a reasonably solid object—when imagining a body jumping on a trampoline, the discussion focused only on stretching of the trampoline alone. But actually the body is also being "displaced"—stretched and moved—when it lands on the trampoline. The skeleton is analogous to the grains of sand, with each bone being moved in a different way through the interaction of gravity, momentum, and ground reaction force. In the human body, however, the bones are held together by elastic tissue, the myofascia, which absorbs the forces coming from each of these three dynamics. This, as you will see, is vital to our understanding of walking, and we must be able to visualize the interactions between the forward momentum of the gait, the downward force of gravity, and the supporting ground reaction forces.

The interaction between the foot and the ground is simple when one is standing still. But in walking, the ground reaction force is not perpendicular to gravity. It is this angle of impact that invokes the folding of the joints throughout the body, and, as we will see as we progress through the book, it is the controlled adjustment of the joints that "loads" the tissue to assist recovery and recoil. (The springs of the trampoline can be seen as an analogy. They are stretched—"loaded" with recoil power—when someone jumps on the trampoline.)

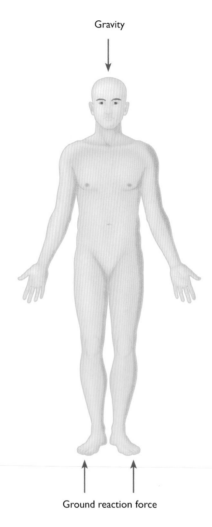

Gravity

Ground reaction force

Figure 1.4. When one is standing quietly, gravity is pulling the center of gravity down, and this is being "met" by the ground reaction force pushing straight up.

A full exploration of ground reaction force gets much more complicated than we need for our overall picture of the economy and cooperation of walking (and it can sprout lots of scary-looking equations), but a simple version of how ground reaction force works will help us see what happens in the body when it interacts with the ground.

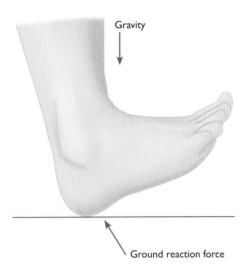

Figure 1.5. As the heel hits the floor, the force "pushes" back at the heel in the opposite direction; this is what decelerates movement of the calcaneus.

ENERGY CONSERVATION

So much of my travelling is done on foot, that if I cherished betting propensities, I should probably be found registered in sporting newspapers under some such title as the Elastic Novice, challenging all eleven stone mankind to competition.
—Charles Dickens, "Shy Neighbourhoods"

Evolution and Economy

Walking upright is one of the factors that sets us apart from our nonhuman primate cousins and is considered to be one of the main forces behind our evolution into our current *Homo sapiens* selves. Creating a stable, resilient form with the least calorie usage has been a driving force within nature. Different animals have used different strategies to achieve this equilibrium; evolution is a multifactorial process that cannot be tied down to any one dynamic. Compare the lumbering gait of a rhinoceros to the waddle of the penguin and to the flow of Grace Kelly's dancing. All are the products of millions of years of evolution on different branches of the tree of life. The rhino has sacrificed grace for strength and a tough hide, allowing it to win most fights in the search for calories. The penguin may look comical on land but is bullet-like in the water, where it meets both its prey and its predators.

Homo sapiens gave up strength and speed and instead aimed for efficiency and generalization. Minimizing our calorie expenditure in the search for food—and maximizing the many strategies we can use to catch, find, or grow it—led to what and where we are now. We made use of many factors inherent in our bodies, especially the potential that was unleashed when we became capable of standing, walking, and running on two legs.

As a nation we are dedicated to keeping physically fit—and parking as close to the stadium as possible.
—Bill Vaughan

Our brain requires sixteen times more energy than the chemical-to-mechanical-energy-transformers we call "muscles." With 20 percent to 25 percent of our daily resources being diverted to the brain, it makes sense that we take measures to ensure the supply of food to this important organ. The current strategy of the average American is to keep bodily exertion to a minimum—for instance, by walking only 350 intermittent yards per day (McCredie 2007). But this is not a good strategy. Strolling short distances, starting and stopping, takes more muscular effort than sustained walking at a regular pace.

Efficiency is of vital importance for our survival: if we can minimize our calorie output and maximize our intake, we are more likely to survive. Any variation in our anatomy that will enhance that ratio in our favor will be more likely to be passed onto the next generation—it will be favorably selected. As Cochran and Harpending demonstrate in their entertaining text *The 10,000 Year Explosion*, genetic changes can spread throughout a population surprisingly quickly, with a natural tendency to favor the more effective or positive influences (2010). For example, they argue that the protein dystrophin may have influenced our ratio of muscle to brains and that the changes in this ratio were selected in a relatively short period of time. Around a hundred thousand years ago, we clearly had more muscle and less brain, but in a relatively short space of time, the amount of energy invested in our brains compared to that invested in our muscles became more balanced. (Though, as we will see in chapter 4, Neanderthals actually had larger brains than we do today.)

Our nonhuman primate cousins have evolved a variety of movement strategies, including the knuckle walking of gorillas and chimpanzees and the four-limbed tree walking of orangutans. Nearly all of them, however, have to use a variation of the bent hip/bent knee posture for movement. This is not due to limitations in length of the hip or knee flexors but rather is caused by a limitation in the lumbar spine, which does not allow for enough extension to bring the pelvis in line with the knees and the feet (see fig. 1.6).

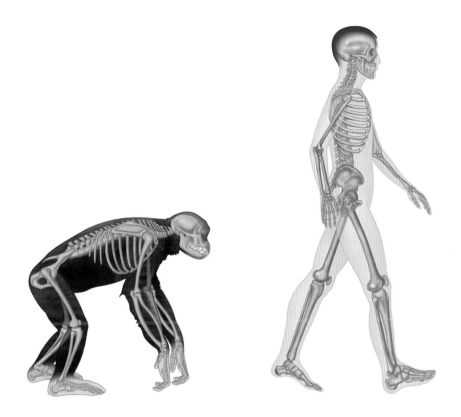

Figure 1.6. It is the lumbar-extension capability of the human that allows the secondary curves of the spine to adapt to an upright stance. This brings the head, thorax, pelvis, knees, and feet into a more vertical alignment.

One effect of the upright stance has been to greatly reduce the size of the spinal erectors, which are in almost constant use in the forward-leaning posture of the other hominids (see fig. 1.7). The cost, however, has been to place the lumbars in a more unstable position, prone to spondylolisthesis and scoliosis (Lovejoy, in Vleeming et al 2007). At first, this may not have been a costly adaptation, as hunter-gatherers may not have lived long enough for these degenerative issues to develop as often as they do today.

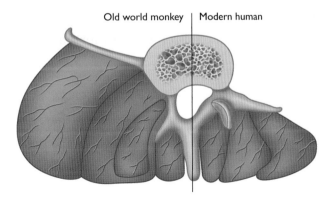

Old world monkey | Modern human

Figure 1.7. Without the constant need for resistance of flexion, the human spinal erectors have a greatly reduced circumference compared to those of the old world monkey (note that the illustration here is a "hybrid" of various species). We can also see how the transverse processes of the human spine are more posteriorly placed, allowing for greater stability in extension, since they are behind the center of the intervertebral discs.

Another important skeletal change in our progression to bipedalism was to bring the ilia into a more lateral orientation. This allows the hip abductors to stabilize the pelvis—in other words, the hip abductors stop us from falling sideways when we stand on one leg (remember, we are on one foot during 80 percent of walking). In all other primates, the ilia face posteriorly, and their hip abductors, especially gluteus maximus and medius, function more as extensors (to push them forward) and give little contribution to lateral stability. This means that they are less able to stand on one leg, an essential part of bipedal gait.

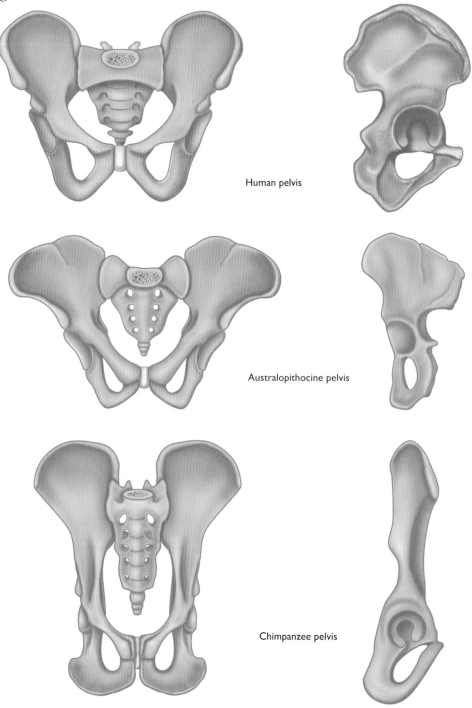

Human pelvis

Australopithocine pelvis

Chimpanzee pelvis

A

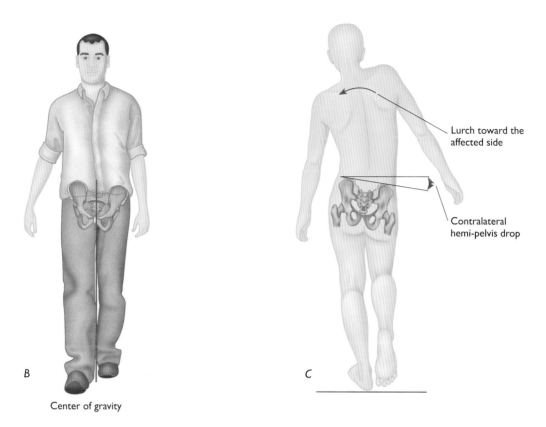

Center of gravity

Figure 1.8. As the ilia of the nonhuman primate face posteriorly (A), the fascicular direction of the hip muscles will be more dominant in the sagittal plane, making them work as extensors of the hip, unlike the laterally oriented human ilia (B). When the gluteal muscles are attached at the side of the body, they are able to support the pelvis in the frontal plane and prevent it from falling to one side. Failure of these muscles demonstrates itself in the Trendelenburg gait (C), in which the pelvis falls significantly to one or both sides.

Much debate exists about what makes us "human"—intelligence, language, cooperation, society, opposable thumbs, and so forth—but many people believe bipedalism was the main mechanism for accelerating our evolution as a race. It freed our hands to manipulate tools and to communicate with gesture. Our comparative muscular weakness and our long period of immaturity in childhood demanded better communication, as well as protection and cooperation in group activities, such as hunting. According to Richard Wrangham, the freedom afforded to our hands through our ability to remain upright allowed us to control fire, giving us the unique ability to cook (2009). The preliminary breakdown of food in cooking increases the availability of calories, as less energy is required during digestion. Therefore, we absorb more fuel from the food we eat, making it easier to feed the resource-demanding brain.

The truth is that there is no one factor that led to us becoming human, but the common factor in most of the theories is that we developed strategies to become more efficient. The changes that occurred within our body mechanics permit a high degree of efficiency, which, as Bramble and Lieberman have shown, allowed us to become persistence hunters, chasing our prey to death (2004). In addition, we were able to take advantage of our reduced stomach size (due to cooking our food?), our enhanced thermoregulation (we sweat more than other animals), our greater breathing capacity, and, last but not least, our elastic fascial efficiency.

The changes that occurred in our skeletal alignment allowed us to use gravity and ground reaction forces to great advantage, giving us a more efficient interaction between our anatomy and the forces around it. We see this when we compare the penguin's waddle and an elegant human gait. We don't always recognize the mechanics involved in those differences though, and this will be the further focus of this book: the synergetic alignment of joints, forces and tissue.

Myofascial Design and the Anatomy Trains

The eccentric lengthening of the tissue that is created by the need for shock absorption also helps the body return in the opposite direction, just like the springs of the trampoline. The myofascia is mechanically loaded, like springs, through the momentum created by the forward and rotational forces of walking, as well as by the pull of gravity. This is performed through relatively passive mechanisms (rather than through muscle contraction) that allow the elastic fascial tissue to be put under stretch in all three planes of motion. Due to the angles and positions of the joints in the body, these forces are not restricted to single muscles—they pass through long, continuous chains of myofascia, most often following the lines of "Anatomy Trains," as put forward by Thomas Myers (2009).

After teaching anatomy for many years within the Rolf Institute, Myers began to see that when the network of connective tissue is examined together with muscle fiber direction, one sees continuous lines of force production throughout the body. He first published his "map" of these Anatomy Trains in 1997 and showed how, when the fascial tissue is stretched over joints, it can transfer force across the joint from one myofascial unit to another. When the joints are in midrange, the tissue is relaxed and communication is limited to the single units on one side of the joint (see exercise 1.1), but in certain stretched positions, closer to the end of range, force transmission is facilitated along the myofascial lines across the joints.

Exercise 1.1. First, extend your wrist and fingers to feel the stretch and then compare the sensation and range of motion when you repeat the wrist extension with your elbow also extended. Finally, draw you arm back and into horizontal abduction, keep your elbow extended and again extend your wrist. Each of these movements will engage more tissue across each subsequent joint. They may or may not affect the range of motion, but the sensations should differ as one brings into play more of what Myers refers to as the Superficial Front Arm Line.

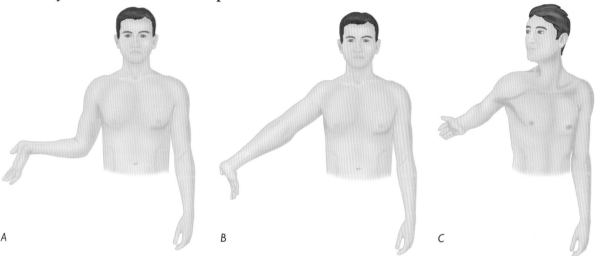

A   B   C

Figure 1.9. By engaging the tissues across the wrist (A), then elbow (B), and finally the gleno-humeral joints (C), each wrist extension will feel differently as more of the Superficial Front Arm Line is brought into the movement. Experiment further by changing the position and angle of the humerus and noticing the effect on the stretch of the wrist flexors. You may find there is a certain angle and position that feels as if it includes the whole of the line. It is this mechanism—the proper positioning that engages the full myofascial line—that we wish to exploit in walking.

When longer myofascial lines are engaged, one part of the body can affect another. Just as the shoulder position affects the hand and wrist in exercise 1.1, so too will the pelvis affect the foot; and the head, the thorax. By visualizing these continuous lines of force through the body, we can interpret the effects of one part on another, understanding how, for example, the shoulder position may affect the tracking of the knee. This will, hopefully, lead to ways of correcting inefficiencies in walking.

Just as we need to consider both the voluntary action and the involuntary reflex reactions of the myofascial system to understand walking, so too do we have to see the myofascial system in terms of both individual muscles and long continuous chains of linked myofascial units. These chains, called "lines" or "Anatomy Trains," allow a long section of the body—rather than, say, an individual muscle in the leg—to contribute to shock absorption and its control, and this provides longer elastic chains that absorb kinetic energy and then recoil with elastic force, thereby allowing for greater energy conservation (see fig. 1.10, overleaf).

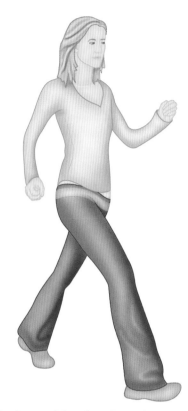

Figure 1.10. At heel strike on the right side, the downward force from the trunk creates a tilt of the pelvis to the left side. This "acceleration" (the sudden tilting to the left) will be perceived and controlled by the hip abductors on the right—the side of heel strike—and the lateral abdominals on the left. Neither the contraction nor the fascial loading will be restricted to just those named muscles, but will go farther along what Myers has named the "Lateral Line."

Myers built this Anatomy Trains model on previous and similar work done by earlier anatomists—such as Dart, Vleeming, and Busquet. He charted a comprehensive map of the biomechanical chains through the body. His work focused on the posture of a person standing still, and initially, the fuller implications of Anatomy Trains in movement were less appreciated. But when we analyze the interactions between gravity and ground reaction force, the continuity of the myofascial system really comes to life. This system lets us track the forces involved in the body in each plane of motion and at differing layers of the body. The Anatomy Trains also show us the tension-adjusting system that helps to disperse the forces the body is exposed to—spreading the "shock" and also, vitally, recruiting distant areas to assist in recovery. This interrelationship of the disparate parts of the body is our key to efficiency, and its understanding helps us to visualize the "walking system."

Tensegrity

We can now begin to see the interplay between the strength and stability of the skeletal system and the adaptability, buoyancy, and tension abilities of the myofascial system. This new model of the human body gives us a way of understanding these integrated systems and how they collaborate to distribute tension and organize response. "Tensegrity" is at play every time we move; it is inherent within our body as far down as the cellular level, but there are few everyday expressions of it more tangible than the poetic, full-body movement of walking.

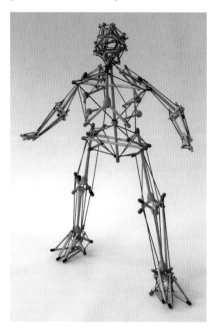

Figure 1.11. When we see the body represented as a tensegrity system like this, with just the musculoskeletal elements presented (in vague approximation of reality), it is easier to comprehend how the body interacts with its environment to dissipate and produce force.

The use of solid elements (bone) and elastic elements (myofascia) requires the presence of a certain amount of prestress. It is the contribution of "tension" that gives the structure "integrity" (and it is the combination of these two words that Fuller used to coin the term *tensegrity*).

One of the characteristics of tensegrity structures is their ability to distribute stress or changes in tension throughout the whole of the structure. This can be either a positive or negative thing, depending on the nature of the change. Too much tension will lead to an increase in stiffness and possible breakdown, while a decrease in tension can cause the structure to lose some of its integrity. Balanced tension allows resilience in the system, giving it the ability to disperse, communicate, and store forces across itself and still maintain equilibrium. This is the essence of what therapists aim to achieve when intervening with a patient's gait: we first need to recognize the imbalance or inability to communicate mechanical force, and then, by appropriate intervention, bring the patient's system to resilience.

While there is some debate over the full application of tensegrity in biological structures, there does seem to be an ever-increasing amount of acceptance of the concept. Tensegrity gives us a framework to explain many aspects of human and animal movement. In doing so, we have come full circle, once again using the understanding of architectural structure and geometry to describe human form.

Don Ingber, a researcher at Harvard Medical School, was the first to apply this new geometrical concept to the body, beginning in the 1980s. Ingber showed how cellular structure and mechanics can be explained through tensegrity. Cells have their own inner supports, which allow the transfer of mechanical forces. These forces can communicate cell shape to the nucleus and thereby influence cellular expressions (Ingber 1998).

Steven Levin, a retired orthopedic surgeon, took this a step further and demonstrated that the pelvic and shoulder girdles and the knee joint are using similar engineering principles. He argues that tensegrity is the essential building mechanism at the level of the cell, the tissues, and the entire body. Adding to Ingber's ideas on the laws of self-assembly (the ways in which the cells combine), many consider that tensegrity elements will follow their natural mechanics and attach to one another to grow ever more complex communities, all following the principles of "tensional integrity."

The sacrum is often illustrated as a keystone that gives the pelvis a compressional locking force, using the cumulative weight of the bones from above to hold the pelvis together. Alternatively, it is described as acting like an arrowhead that would split the two sides of the pelvis apart. When the pelvis is examined in cross section (see fig. 1.12), however, the sacrum is clearly shown to be suspended between the ilia. It therefore helps draw the two sides of the pelvis together, using tension from the myofascial guide-wires. In chapter 5, "Spiral Line," we will see that the "flotation" of the sacrum between the ilia is essential in mediating the many forces that come from the upper and lower bodies. The sacroiliac joints act as a hub for force mediation through the pelvis.

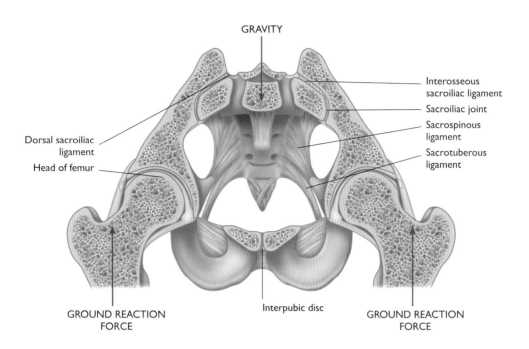

Figure 1.12.When seen in cross section, it is clear that the sacrum is suspended from the ilia, like a hammock between the trees of the ilia; the dorsal sacroiliac ligaments are akin to the ropes of the hammock. Levin argues that the sacrum has to act within the joints to mediate the various forces coming from above and below—gravity and ground reaction force. Furthermore, he argues that the sacrum is supported in the tension created by the "approximation" force (the force that draws two sides together) of the dorsal sacroiliac ligaments, rather than by the compression of the ilia.That is, it is a tensegrity structure (in Vleeming et al 2007).

As discussed above, any force applied to a tensegrity structure is dispersed through its entirety, and when we look more closely at distortion, we see two very important phenomena. The first is that tension elements align themselves along the line of pull, helping to increase resistance along that line—effectively making the structure stiffer (and therefore stronger) as more lines are recruited to oppose the stress. This is an important feature of many biological tissues—they get stiffer under stress, meaning that the stronger the force, the more resistance they have.

A second characteristic of tensegrity structures is that once the strain is removed, the structure returns to its normal resting balance. Tensegrity structures are therefore self-supporting, not requiring the addition of gravity to maintain or hold their form (compared to a tower of blocks, which requires the compression of gravity and loses all integrity when turned at an angle to gravity). Tensegrity structures have an internal resilience that absorbs the energy of external forces and then uses it to return to neutral. The human body applies this dynamic in efficient walking, using the interaction of momentum, gravity, and the resistance from the ground to tension the tissues, and as the body position changes, this tension is released to assist with the return movement, somewhat like a watch-spring mechanism.

TRIANGULATION

By standing upright, humans have taken fuller advantage of one of tensegrity's dynamic characteristics. We are less stable by having only two contact points with the ground, and we further exacerbate that instability by balancing on one leg during 80 percent of walking and 100 percent of running (excluding the flight phase of running, when we have no contact with the ground). To manage this acrobatic act, we have changed the way in which the forces pass through the body, allowing for much more three-dimensional variation.

In the tensegrity of the upright body, the compression elements (the bones) are supported by the elastic, tensioning forces (the myofascia). The vectors of support are arranged in a triangulated pattern following mathematical laws similar to those of crystal formation. As Levin shows, a triangular truss is much more able to disperse force within itself than a square frame (in Vleeming et al 2007, see fig. 1.13). This is important to keep in mind, as the body rarely uses movement in just one plane of motion, making it difficult to track events as we go through a movement. Tension is created in each plane: frontal, sagittal, and transverse. I will simplify this in the book by dealing with each in turn, but they are all acting simultaneously.

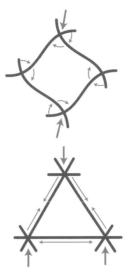

Figure 1.13. A square-based arrangement will tend to buckle under stress, compared to a triangulated structure, which is able to deal with both compression and tension along its axis.

When tensions in the body are balanced, there is a sense of effortlessness; the bones are "floating in a sea of tension," as Myers said, and any changes in that equilibrium will be easily absorbed and recoiled back with the natural resilience of the tissue (2009). It is easy for us to imagine the muscular system as the controllers of this tensioning, but the muscles are only one element of the supportive tissues that hold the bones in place. The primary tissues of the system are the fascial tissues. The muscles are essentially the fine tuners of the system, adding or subtracting tension when needed, via the fascial tissues of the body.

FASCIAL MEMBRANES

As mentioned earlier, each and every part of the body is wrapped within the fibrous, fascial web of connective tissue, which consists predominantly of collagen, elastin, and ground substance (a gel-like fluid consisting of water along with various sugars and proteins). The fascia holds each and every part of our body together and it provides us with protection, both mechanical and chemical—the fascia forms a physical barrier, and the fluid within the fascia contains many lymphocytes. The fibrous elements allow the transfer of force (created either by muscle contractions or external forces), but they do so with an element of elasticity, which gives us the "spring in our step." This pliability is enhanced through the engagement of longer lines of tissue, the connections of one myofascial unit to another and another, such as those felt in exercise 1.1.

Force is most often considered in terms of straight lines, along muscle fibers and out into tendons and ligaments. This bias is inherent within the presentations of the Anatomy Train lines, but it is a misunderstanding, as we need to regard fascial aponeuroses and consider that the Anatomy Trains are communicating through these tissues as well.

Many of the fascial wrapping sheaths in the body are extensions of muscular tissue. These often play an important role in dispersing force by acting as "hydraulic amplifiers" (Gracovetsky 2008; DeRosa and Porterfield in Vleeming et al 2007). To understand a "hydraulic amplifier," imagine the example of a balloon. The tension of the outer rubber membrane and the compression of the air inside it create a "stiffening" dynamic within the structure. If the balloon is not fully inflated, however, there will be little tension created on the outside. The balloon will be less resilient and will mold itself to the surface it is resting on, rather than being independently buoyant on it. Conversely, if the balloon is overinflated, the rubber becomes fatigued and will lose its ability to adapt to the tension—it will burst. In the fascia, the body's encasing material, similar events can occur.

This has been studied primarily in the thoracolumbar and thigh areas, where the muscles of the pelvis and the lower back are dealing with high stress loads in various vectors of force and at different anatomical depths (see fig. 1.14, overleaf). In cross section, we can see the continuity of the posterior and middle layers of the thoracolumbar fascia wrapping around the muscles—stabilizing, supporting, or moving the lower back.

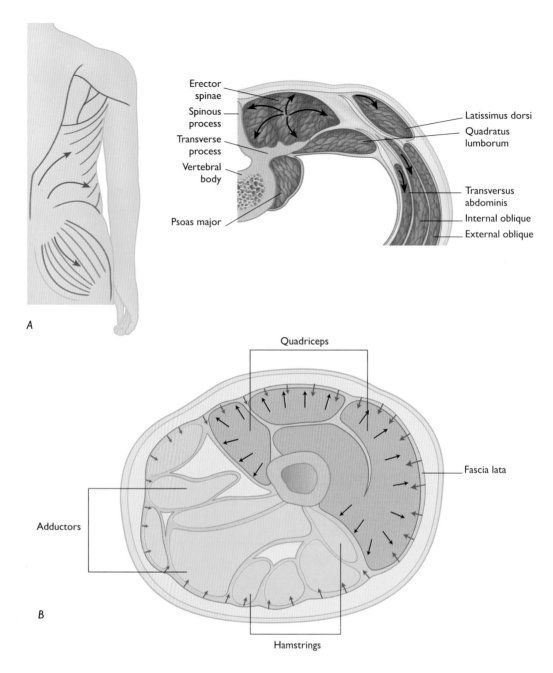

Figure 1.14 In walking, the thoracolumbar fascia will be tensioned by the contralateral contraction of the gluteus maximus and latissimus dorsi. This creates tension in the supporting fascia around the lower back muscles, which in turn "pump up" the fascia by pushing out against it when they contract to support the spine. This creates a force-dispersal system and is a mechanism used in various parts of the body, including the thigh (B). The enveloping fascia of the thigh, the fascia lata, is tensioned by the appropriately named tensor fascia lata and by the gluteus maximus. Both of those muscles are, in fact, encased within that layer of fascial tissue. This inward force is then matched by the outward expansion of the underlying muscles, which will be contracting to support the knee and hip.

In walking, there is tensioning of the gluteus maximus and latissimus dorsi muscles, which are connected via the thoracolumbar fascia. This fascial sheet and its deeper connections will therefore be tensioned, like the skin of a balloon, and this "shrink wrapping" force will meet the expansion of the muscles within it, creating a taut "balloon" capable of easy force transfer and recoil. It is estimated that this form of hydraulic amplifier can increase the efficiency of muscle contractions by up to 30 percent, though if the fascial sheets are challenged, as in a fasciotomy (the cutting of the fascia to relieve underlying pressure), efficiency can be decreased by 10 percent to 16 percent (Parker and Briggs 2007).

All of these myofascial layers, while separate in terms of depth and the forces they carry, are connected to one another by a different kind of fluid-rich fascial tissue, known as "areolar" or "loose connective" tissue. This tissue provides the lubrication within the system that enables each plane to glide on its neighbor. This tissue can sometimes can be prone to changes in local hydration, creating adhesions which inhibit the relative movement between the different planes.

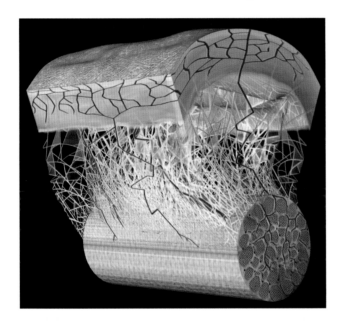

Figure 1.15. The very fluid areolar tissue contains collagen and elastin fibers, like fascia, but within a much higher concentration of ground substance. This compliant tissue connects fascial layers and facilitates movement by adapting its orientation to the vector of forces involved.
Reproduced with the kind permission of Dr J.C. Guimberteau and EndovivoProductions.

STIFFNESS

Stiffness, not the early-morning type of stiffness that increases with age, but rather the tissues' resistance to deformation, is an essential feature of the body. The body's skeletal structure is inherently unstable, and each bone interfaces with another on curved surfaces. One role of the soft tissue is to give resistance, or stiffness, to the system, to ensure that it doesn't collapse under the pressure of external forces.

It does this in a number of different ways. First, there is the mechanical influence of the collagen and elastin fibers that hold everything in place (see fig. 1.16). Both types of fiber are "elastic," able to stretch beyond their normal resting length and then return to their original resting length. Elastin is able to lengthen more than the collagen, but collagen, when stretched, will recoil back to its neutral with more efficiency. What this means is that collagen is truly more "elastic" than elastin, as it gives more elastic energy back into the system.

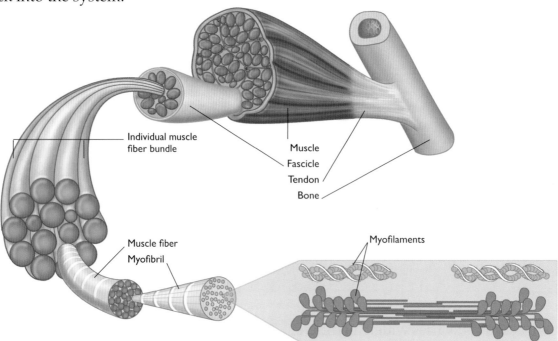

Figure 1.16. Each muscle is encased within a series of fascial bags—the epimysium, perimysium, and endomysium—which are made up of various types of collagen fiber, with a blend of elastin and the more-fluid ground substance.

To explain the importance of this, we need to look at normal movement. A number of experiments have shown that during repetitive movements such as walking, there is very little change in the length of the muscle fibers, which are often used in *isometric* contraction (i.e., they are not becoming shorter when they contract—they are simply maintaining their current length, see fig. 1.17). The lengthening required during walking actually occurs in the fascial tissues, in the collagen and elastin, which are able to recoil from the stretch and return to their resting length, like a spring.

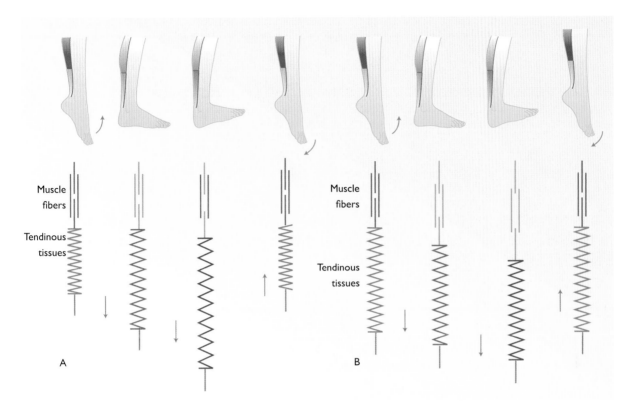

Figure 1.17. In this diagram, the fascial tissue is represented as the "elastic" tissue (using Hookean springs) and the contractile muscle as sliding filaments. In a series of experiments, Fukunaga and colleagues showed that in cyclical movements the muscles tended to remain predominately isometric (A) rather than doing the extra work on concentric and eccentric contraction (B), 2002 and 2006.

The main benefit of this arrangement is that the recoil of the fascial tissue is providing essentially free energy. The fascia is stretched by the body's momentum and its interaction with the ground. If the actin and myosin filaments (the sliding elements within the muscle fibers that control contraction) do not allow the muscle to lengthen, then the forces involved in movement have to be absorbed by the fibrous tissue. The fascial tissue is transforming kinetic energy into potential energy by absorbing energy and then releasing it back into the system as kinetic energy again. It is impossible to give exact figures for the amount of stretch and recoil that is produced in each fascial tissue, because it varies widely in different parts of the body, but it can be as much as 93 percent of the energy being given back into the system (McNeill Alexander 2002).

Once again, we see the body's drive for efficiency come into play. The active concentric and eccentric contraction of muscles is expensive, requiring the exchange of adenosine triphosphate (ATP) and glucose. Much less fuel is required when muscle fibers are held in isometric contraction. One of the hallmarks of efficient walking is the absence of active muscular contraction, maximizing the recoil efficiency of the fascial tissues; an easy walking pattern should use only around 38 percent of the body's maximal aerobic capacity.

FASCIAL EFFICIENCY

I can remember walking as a child. It was not customary to say you were fatigued. It was customary to complete the goal of the expedition.
—Katharine Hepburn

What the role of fascia in walking means is that we need to change how we think about muscles. The old idea of movement via concentric, eccentric, and occasional isometric contraction is just not how the body works in many functions. The muscles work as a stiffness adjusting system. Just as a Pilates instructor changes the springs on a reformer to suit the client or the exercise, so too does the neuromyofascial system adjust the springs to match the forces in the tissue, a constant computational task and one that we still fail to fully understand.

As discussed above, the body needs something to hold it together; it is a bag of bones that, due to their slippery ends, require additional support from the surrounding tissue. The joints—the interfaces between the bones—fold, bend, flex, rotate, or extend in predictable directions. They are therefore able to guide the forces in the body: when the quadriceps contracts, the force is transmitted via the patella to extend the knee. However, when we look at the interaction between the body and the ground, the relationship is reversed: it is the bending of the knee on impact that sends the force to the quadriceps, sparking its contraction.

This reversal of function is important. When we look at movements involving some form of impact with a surface, it is the channeling effect of the joint that creates the movement, not the muscle. The joints are like dry riverbeds that direct the water through the landscape via the path of least resistance. Any movement that creates a normal impact on the body, such as heel strike in walking, will require the deceleration of momentum (and I will outline the many ways the body does this in the next chapter by tracing the action across the major joints involved in walking).

Using the conventional eccentric/concentric contractions of muscles for each step would require a large amount of resources. The body would have to constantly bind and unbind the actin and myosin filaments of the muscles. We often feel the effects of this muscular type of movement when we go for strolls involving a lot of stopping and starting, such as meandering around a museum or shopping with loved ones on a Saturday afternoon. The constant stopping and starting requires more muscular effort and is therefore much more tiring than going for a long, evenly paced walk, which allows other, more efficient mechanisms to come into play.

In the repetitive motions of walking, the inner tuning of our springs is unconscious. Apparently even the spinal cord is rarely involved in controlling the movement—it is the local relationship between the mechanoreceptors in the fascial tissue and the surrounding "adjusters" of the muscles that are in charge. By finding the most efficient level of stiffness, the body can maximize the use of elastic recoil and minimize the metabolic costs.

Deformation and Elasticity

Could the young but realize how soon they will become mere walking bundles of habits, they would give more heed to their conduct while in the plastic state.
—William James

As we saw in the Fukunaga experiments reported above (see fig. 1.17), the force-guiding effect of the joints will lead to *deformation* of the myofascia in repetitive motions such as walking. *Deformation* is defined as any compression, shear, or tension. I will concentrate on the production of tension that creates stress in the tissues and thereby lengthens them. The amount the tissues lengthen depends on a number of factors, including age, hydration, and nutrition, but it also depends on the quality of that tissue, as not all myofascia is the same. Some myofascia will have more connective tissue, and this will affect its elasticity (its ability to lengthen and return to its original position). For example, there is an obvious difference in the architecture of the gastrocnemius, the sartorius, and the semimembranosus (see fig. 1.18, overleaf). The passive force curve (which measures the elasticity of the connective tissue in each muscle) illustrates the greater stiffness of the gastrocnemius and shows how its resistance to stretch begins sooner than in the sartorius or semimembranosus. This means that the connective tissue of the gastrocnemius is stretched earlier in its movement, and it requires more energy to be lengthened, an important feature for economy of gait.

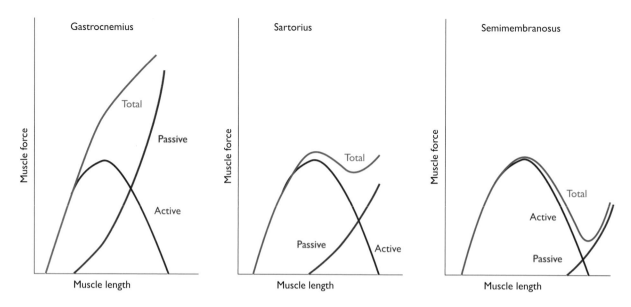

Figure 1.18. Based on work done by Wilkie in 1968, Komi (2011) points out that the gastrocnemius has shorter fascicles, which means that it will be less able to stretch than the longer-fibered thigh muscles of sartorius and semimembranosus. This will send the force of that stretch into gastrocnemius's connective tissue at a shorter range of motion (the gastrocnemius has more connective tissue for this reason). Areas of the body with higher mechanical stress will use a number of strategies to deal with the extra loading. One of those is a greater amount of connective tissue, which protects the area and allows the force to be absorbed and returned as energy. We will also see later that the pennation, in which the muscle fibers attach to the tendon at an oblique angle, adds efficiency to this system.

By elongating the connective tissue of the gastrocnemius, for example, we are creating a store of energy. Most organic materials have some form or amount of elastic ability; they are able to stretch (deform) and then return to their original length. The obvious example is a rubber band, which requires work to stretch but then will recoil to its original state by itself. If you pull a rubber band, you feel the energy required to stretch it, and if it snaps back against your fingers, you will certainly experience the energy available in the return. In the case of the body's movement in walking, the elastic tissue is stretched ("loaded") quite passively, through the natural pressure of gravity and ground reaction force.

The amount of energy returned with the recoil does not always match that which created it (some energy is lost in the system), but in terms of economy, connective tissue is quite efficient: up to 93 percent of energy is returned to the system. This means that a lot of the energy being used in walking is almost "free"—it does not require the active contraction of the muscles and the use of oxygen. Some measurements have calculated that about 17 percent of the force required in running comes from the recoil of the arches of the feet, and 16 percent of walking from the Achilles tendon (Blazevich 2011).

The loss of energy from the system is referred to as *hysteresis* (see fig. 1.19). Some energy loss is due to the *viscosity* of the tissue, which is its resistance to deformation. This varies considerably, depending on the chemical nature and make-up of the tissues involved, all of which can also create slight delay in tissue recoil.

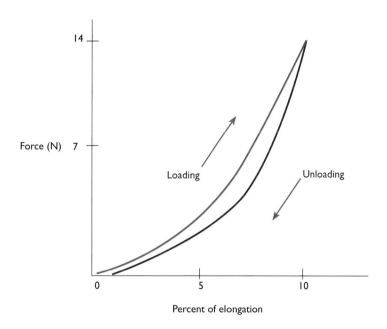

Figure 1.19. The graph illustrates the nonlinear nature of the amount of force required to stretch connective tissue (i.e., more force is required for the second centimeter of stretch than was needed for the first). The blue line maps the tissue's elastic return to resting length. In a truly efficient system, the two lines would match (i.e., the same force would return to the system). The gap between the two lines illustrates the lost energy due to hysteresis, an inherent property of the tissue.

Viscoelasticity

The viscosity within the connective tissue is a double-edged sword: while it robs us of some of the available recoil energy, it also absorbs a portion of the body's momentum, particularly in its struggle against gravity, and by doing so, it removes some of the workload from the muscles. Connective tissue is often referred to as *viscoelastic* because of this combination of properties.

The fluid element within fascia, the ground substance, is made up of proteins and sugars (glycosaminoglycans) and behaves in a nonlinear fashion. Sometimes referred to as a non-Newtonian fluid (so-called because it does not react to forces in a linear, "Newton-approached" fashion), the ground substance can become "stickier" and, when force is applied at speed, can provide more stiffness for the system.

You may have felt this reaction when comparing a Hatha yoga–type slow stretch to a plyometric exercise. The sharper, faster movements of the plyometrics create a strong and often linear response in the tissue compared to movement entered into slowly, which has a more dispersed effect. The viscosity can be affected by a number of factors, including heat (compare a Bikram yoga class to stretching at the North Pole) and the hydration of the tissue (the ground substance is extremely hydrophilic and needs to bind to water molecules to maintain fluidity). This mechanism comes into play during walking: when a joint is encouraged to move in the deceleration phase—after heel strike, when the system is working to absorb the force of gravity and the ground reaction force—the viscous ground substance will stiffen the tissue and thereby allow the fascial fibers to load more, taking further advantage of the elastic recoil.

Stretch Reflex

The elastic stretching of the tissue also stimulates many of the body's mechanoreceptors, the proprioceptors for the body. The muscle spindle, in particular, sensing the stretch within the myofascia, will set off the stretch reflex arc (see fig. 1.20).

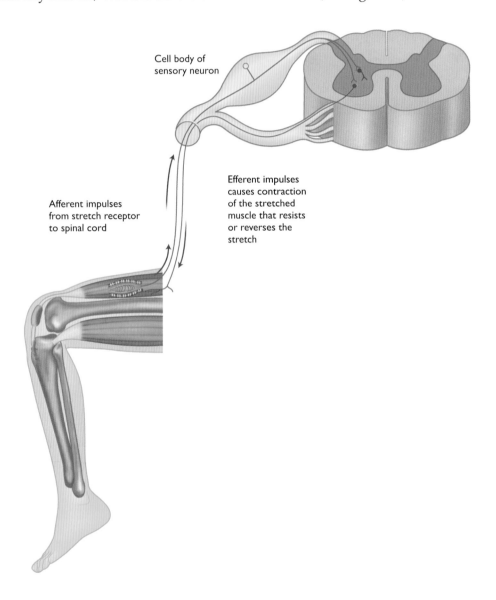

Cell body of
sensory neuron

Efferent impulses
causes contraction
of the stretched
muscle that resists
or reverses the
stretch

Afferent impulses
from stretch receptor
to spinal cord

Figure 1.20. The lengthening of the myofascia is sensed by the muscle spindle, which signals the spinal cord. The spinal cord responds with an efferent (motor) nerve signal for the muscle to contract.

The reflex arc creates the contraction of the muscle, which is predominately isometric. Further deceleration of the body's movement then loads the connective tissue, which eventually reaches a point at which the force required to lengthen it farther has been absorbed by the increasing stiffness of the elastic fiber. Once it reaches the point at which the force stretching the fiber equals the tension within it, it begins to recoil, just like a weight bouncing on the end of a spring. The amount of energy lost by the system can depend on the period of time spent at the end of range. This *amortization, or transition phase,* will affect the amount of recoil.

Exercise 1.2—Amortization Exercise

These three jumping exercises illustrate the variations and differences in the loading of elastic tissue. Just notice what feels right for your own body, as well as noticing what height you attain with each jump.

A. First try jumping without first bringing your head closer to the floor (i.e., don't bend your knees before the jump). This is difficult, as you will only be able to rely on the power of your ankle plantarflexors. Notice how high you are able to get from the floor with just those muscles.

B. Now bend your knees and stay for a moment in the flexed position before jumping. In this jump, you will be able to take advantage of the power of the hip and knee extensors as well as your lower leg muscles.

C. Finally, bend your knees as in *B,* but jump in a flowing movement, coming down farther, into a squat, and then almost immediately pushing up (as you probably wanted to in jump *A*). You will feel the benefit of the additional elastic recoil.

The jump in *B* added the strong thigh muscles but didn't allow the additional energy of elastic loading, because too much time was spent in the *transition phase.* This is also one of the effects of "museum walking": the stop-and-start nature of it takes away the free energy of the elastic tissue. Rhythm is therefore important, and this can be felt in actions such as jumping and hopping: when done too slowly or too quickly the effort becomes muscular, but somewhere in the middle, the movement will take advantage of elastic recoil and will feel "just right."

That is not to say no muscle energy will be involved, just that the ratio will favor elasticity. And, of course, it will also depend on the activity being done and the person's tissue type, as well as which myofascial areas are being tensioned.

Rhythm will influence the amount of energy we can garner from the fascial tissues (as seen in exercise 1.2). This can vary significantly from person to person and will depend on a variety of factors, including tissue type (loosely or tightly ligamented for example), hydration, age, and the general condition of the tissue. A number of experiments have looked at the reasons why we use different types of movement at different speeds. A walk uses a different strategy from a run, and they both differ from a sprint. Studies of energy usage have found that whenever the movement style is changed to match the speed of movement, there is a recovery of efficiency, that is, less energy is used.

Running at a low speed is less efficient than walking, due to the way the tissues are being loaded. This is probably caused by the increased time in the transition phase, because of the longer stride in running increases downward momentum, forcing the muscles to work to recover. Walking with less upward/downward movement compared to running is only efficient up to 7.25 to 7.4 kilometers per hour, at which speed we tend to change to running (McArdle 2010). The increased speed of the run will utilize the up/down loading into the tissue and the amount of time in the transition phase will be reduced. This has been studied in horses, as they change the style of gait from walk to trot to canter and, finally, to gallop. This gradual increase in speed inevitably leads to an increase in muscle work, but with each gait change, there is a recovery of relative efficiency by taking advantage of more elastic energy being returned from the fascial tissue (Biewener 1998).

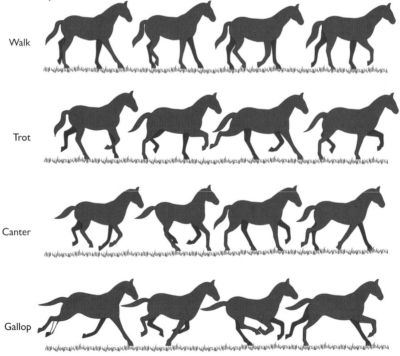

Figure 1.21. Each speed of gait is associated with a different pattern of body use. Changing the length of the stride is one of many strategies to maximize efficiency at each "gear change."

Different movement strategies are used at various speeds to maintain elastic efficiency, but so too must we adapt to other changes in the forces of gravity and ground reaction. Some studies have shown that some African women are able to carry up to 20 percent of their own body weight on their heads and still maintain the same efficiency in walking (Maloiy et al. 1986; McArdle 2010). The analysis of the reasons for this is not fully complete, but it seems that the women are able to transform the increased downward momentum caused by the extra weight into elastic energy rather than muscle effort. We will see how the displacement of body weight can assist elastic loading and recoil throughout the book: vertical displacement predominately loads the Superficial Front and Back Lines, frontal plane movement loads the Lateral Lines, and movement in the transverse plane will affect the Spiral and Functional Lines.

THE STRETCH SHORTENING CYCLE AND WALKING— "EVERY STEP IS A CONTROLLED FALL."

The *stretch shortening cycle* is the basis for many normal human activities, and it utilizes all of the above mechanisms: stretch reflex, elastic recoil, and viscoelasticity. It requires a preparatory movement (or a countermovement) to stimulate the muscle spindles to isometrically contract the muscle, which forces the stretch of the elastic tissues. In walking, this happens through the natural folding of the joints, but in other actions, such as throwing, it is achieved through a countermovement, using the opposite action to load the tissues, often for a movement that will be faster than muscle contraction alone.

Muscle integrity is important, as the muscle must be strong enough to decelerate movement to ensure the fascial tissue is stretched by the momentum. Muscle tendon units do more for the body than simply lengthen and shorten, "they can act as rigid struts to transfer mechanical energy, as a motor to produce mechanical energy, as a damper to dissipate mechanical energy or as a spring to store and return elastic energy" (Sawicki et al. 2009).

All of these roles have to be coordinated. Any loss of elasticity in one area will lead to increased muscle work at another area. For example, imagine losing the ability to plantarflex at push-off, a predominately elastic mechanism. Some other part of the leg would have to compensate for that loss of kinetic energy, most likely a muscle, and that concentric muscle contraction have metabolic costs.

SUMMARY

1. Due to the energy demands of the brain, the human body tries to minimize the amount of calories consumed by muscle work.

2. The development of upright gait freed our hands for other tasks, many of which had calorie-saving or calorie-consuming benefits. This required a number of alterations in our anatomy, which will be outlined in this book.

3. The use of the stretch shortening cycle is our preferred method of motivation in normal everyday movement. The alternative—the constant elongation and shortening of muscles—requires the repeated engagement and release of the actin and myosin elements, which requires a greater use of energy within the body. The stretch shortening cycle eliminates some energy use by taking advantage of three mechanisms: the tissue's viscoelasticity, to begin the deceleration; the stretch reflex, to isometrically contract the muscle tissue; and then the elastic lengthening and recoil of the fascial tissues.

4. Pre-tensioning of myofascial units and elastically loading them through preparatory countermovements adds to the body's mechanical efficiency, decreasing overall metabolic cost as well as increasing the available energy for any single action (such as jumping, as in exercise 1.2).

5. The body has a natural design of myofascial continuities within it, and different movement strategies can incorporate more of them, which will further increase the efficiency of the movement. These "Anatomy Trains" help to disperse force, maximize elastic loading, and use movement of one body segment to facilitate the movement of another.

6. By "triangulating"—using a combination of these lines of force—the body also gains more effective control over movement than it would have if it relied on just one. Incorporating forces from slightly different angles allows for finer control in response to deviating influences.

7. When any part of the body impacts with a surface (most often the foot on the ground), the orientation of the joints serves to send the force of the impact into soft tissue along predictable channels. These channels have presumably adapted over time and serve to spread and absorb the shock; most of them will follow the Anatomy Trains.

8. This predictable order and direction of the folding in the joints then creates the proper conditions to tension the myofascial tissue for greatest economy in their return movement.

Through the rest of the book, I will intermingle elements of comparative anatomy to help visualize the effects of the changes that have occurred in our structure over the course of our evolution. I hope to demonstrate that we need to have a clearer map of the way the body channels kinetic energy and stores it for reuse in the return movement. This first requires an understanding of the events that take place around the joints and bones, and we will then venture into the long myofascial chains that my teacher, Thomas Myers, has referred to as the "Anatomy Trains."

2 The Mechanical Chain

If you seek creative ideas go walking. Angels whisper to a man when he goes for a walk.
—Raymond I. Myers

FUNCTIONS OF WALKING

Perry lists four functions of walking: propulsion, stance stability, shock absorption, and energy conservation (2010). Each of them helps to clarify the role of the soft tissues in walking. We looked at energy conservation in the previous chapter, so we will deal with the first three here.

Propulsion

To understand propulsion, we have to know about both the voluntary and the reflex actions and abilities of the myofascial system, as explained in chapter 1. Much of human movement is goal oriented: we think of a desired outcome, and our body takes us toward it (remember that walking is often a method of getting our head or hands to where we want them). We do not have the space and energy in our conscious minds to sequentially send each and every signal to the relevant musculature. Instead, as demonstrated in the previous chapter, humans allow the somatic nervous system to take over the jobs of initiation and direct propulsion.

As mentioned in chapter 1, the natural folding patterns of the joints sends the force of the movement into the channels of the soft tissue, causing a reaction in the local proprioceptive reflexes embedded and hardwired in the fascial tissue. These reflexes give localized and fast control in response to the mechanics of the tissue around them, thereby reducing the need for signals to be sent all the way up to the spinal cord or—causing even more delay—to the brain and back.

Stance Stability

For us to walk on two legs, we have to be able to stand on one leg, and that depends on our ability to align our center of gravity above our point of contact with the ground. To achieve this, our anatomy has evolved in ways different from that of our primate cousins. The main change is the carrying angle between the hip joint and the knee: the human leg angles inward to allow the feet to align more closely with the midline and the body's center of gravity. In nonhuman primates, there is very little approximation of the knees and feet, meaning that their lower legs lie quite lateral to the line of gravity, making it much more likely that they would fall if they were to stand on one leg (see fig. 2.1).

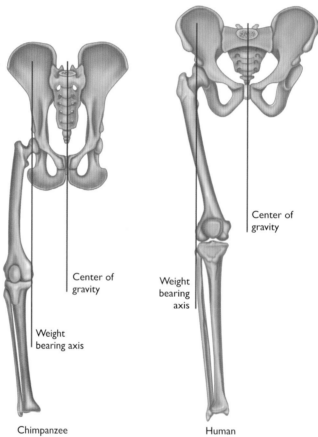

Center of gravity

Weight bearing axis

Center of gravity

Weight bearing axis

Chimpanzee

Human

Figure 2.1. The oblique angle of the human leg allows the support of the body's center of gravity to be brought closer in alignment to its supporting leg. The vertical angle of the primate leg maintains that line of force medial to the support when standing on one leg.

When walking, humans move their feet even closer to the midline, again helping to bring the line of support below the center of gravity. The average separation of the feet is 8 centimeters for men and 7 centimeters for women.

Stability is enhanced in humans by the posterior aspect of the human ilium facing more laterally than that of nonhuman primates, as we saw earlier (see fig. 2.2). The fascicular direction of the gluteal muscles is altered as they cross the lateral midline of the body, and they can therefore act in abducting as well as extending the hip. Abduction—or should we call it "prevention of adduction"?—is vital to the ability to stand on one leg. Much of this angle of support is missing from the nonhuman primate pelvis, which faces posteriorly, making their gluteal muscles primarily extensors—excellent for pushing forward but not great for creating stability in single leg stance.

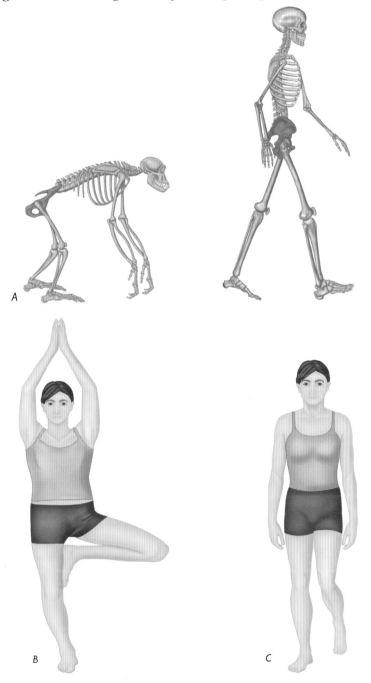

Figure 2.2. A, We can see the alteration in angle, which took place at some point during evolution, that allowed the hip extensors of the nonhuman primate to face more laterally, thereby creating the ability to stand on one leg, an essential part of bipedal gait. B, To achieve and maintain this pose for any length of time, we can see how the carrying angle described above (the medial placement of the knee and, therefore, the foot) and the line of force of contraction from the laterally facing abductors help to keep the body's center of gravity from falling to the left. C, Here we see the necessity for lateral stability, as one leg is in contact with the ground while the other swings through into flexion.

Shock Absorption

The natural rise and fall of human gait creates a force of impact following heel strike that needs to be dissipated before reaching the top of the body in order to keep the head relatively steady. The heel strike of a normal gait pattern produces both an upward and backward need for deceleration. This is where the joints and their alignment with the soft tissue excel.

On impact, the joints will fold naturally, according to the interaction between the ground reaction force, the momentum of the movement, and the location of the body's center of gravity. This natural folding channels the mechanical information about the impact into the "streams" of the soft tissue to be sensed by the proprioceptors encased within the fascia. If the mechanical communication is working, the appropriate muscular forces are activated to prevent collapse.

As we saw above, when looking at ground reaction force, we may need to reverse some of our preconceptions about the joint and muscle interactions. We normally view the active contraction of the muscles—often a conscious or goal-oriented action—as being the motivators of movement across joints, which is the predominant modus operandi in the upper body. This erroneous view is due to the early investigations into muscle actions using electrodes and hooks on lifeless subjects, which did not explore the true interaction of muscles and joints.

When there is a movement in which a force is created through contact with another surface, it is the natural tendency of the joint that will determine the action of the soft tissue, using the myofascial proprioceptors—that is, the action of the soft tissue is a reaction to the joint's movement. For example, you may have been taught to bend your knees when landing after a jump, but in reality, that is all the knee joints can do; their only other choice is to stay straight. The bending of the knee sends the force into the strong quadriceps group, which can act eccentrically to absorb the downward force, decelerating the body (see fig. 2.3).

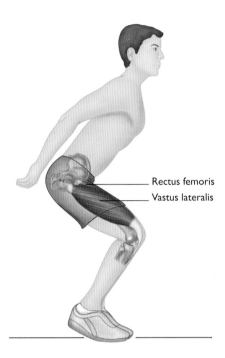

Rectus femoris
Vastus lateralis

Figure 2.3. The knees—and many other joints—can allow the myofascial tissue to absorb much of the force of landing from a jump by collapsing along their predetermined vectors. This channels the mechanical force into soft tissue, which can eccentrically lengthen to decelerate the body.

As we will see in the biomechanical chain, a number of joints will act to absorb the various forces in the three dimensions, not only maintaining equilibrium, but also assisting with the efficiency of movement. The joints determine the vectors of force, which are controlled by the neuromyofascial web and—provided there is the correct stiffness in the surrounding soft tissue—the shock will be absorbed. However, if there is too much mobility or not enough inherent strength in the musculature, there will be a relative collapse of the joint, potentially causing hypermobility of the joint and creating the need for muscles elsewhere to compensate for the loss in elastic energy.

STAGES OF GAIT

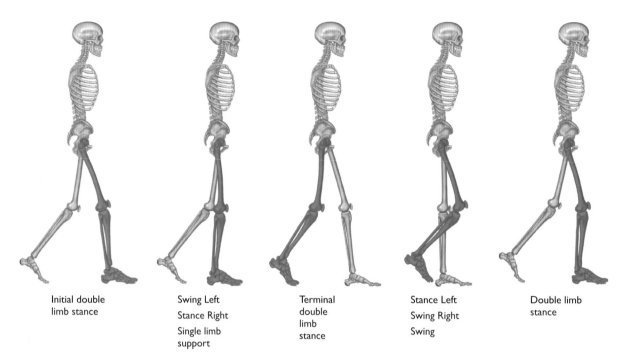

| Initial double limb stance | Swing Left Stance Right Single limb support | Terminal double limb stance | Stance Left Swing Right Swing | Double limb stance |

Figure 2.4. The Stages of Gait (after Perry and Burnfield 2010).

One of the difficulties of analyzing gait has always been the continuous three-dimensional changes. The basic phases are outlined as the Initial Double Limb Stance, Single Limb Support/Swing Phase, Terminal Double Limb Stance, Swing Phase/Single Limb Stance and Double Limb Stance to describe a full stride (two steps).

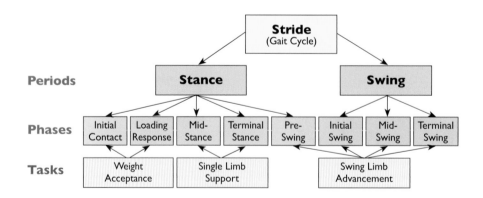

Figure 2.5. Divisions of the gait cycle.

A familiarity with these terms will serve you well, but it is not essential that you remember them now. As you work through the book and understand what is happening at each phase, the terms will become clear.

THE SKELETAL CHAIN

The Joints and Anatomy Trains

It is the balance between mobility and stability—moving enough and not too much—that defines healthy walking. The ability to first see any faults and then intervene with appropriate action is the role of therapist, so as we build the picture of each Anatomy Train's contribution, we will also break it down into a series of "essential events," the things that must occur in each joint to allow the myofascia to properly engage across the joint, enabling the transfer of force in both directions.

The Superficial Back Line is an easy example: when the knee is extended, the tissue of the gastrocnemius and the hamstrings will interact with one another. One can feel this when performing a simple forward bend: the range of motion is greatly increased if it is done with the knees flexed, which unlocks this portion of the line (see fig. 2.6).

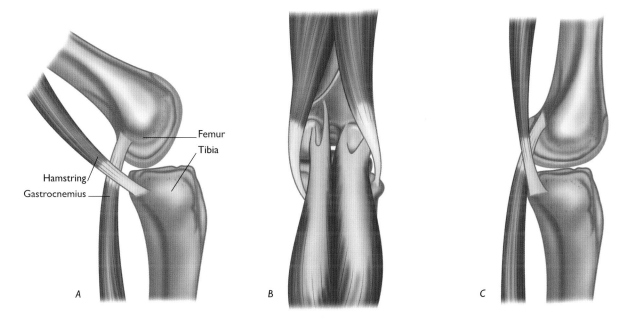

Femur
Tibia
Hamstring
Gastrocnemius

A   B   C

Figure 2.6. When the flexed knee joint (A) comes toward the end of range (B & C), the tissue across the joint becomes aligned and allows the force from one segment to travel to the next. This dynamic can work in any direction, through each of the planes of motion. We will see that this is vital in the creation of myofascial elastic "triggers," which lead to the catapult effect, the release of elastic force to assist with propulsion (see chapter 3). Though the example shown here refers to the knee, the same principle will hold true in the body's other joints as well—to communicate force across them, they must reach a certain degree of motion.

The Anatomy Trains therefore provide us with a map of how the body can transfer mechanical force across body segments when the tissue is allowed to engage. This will require the correct amount of motion at each joint (the "essential events"). And, as we will see, they also provide us with the tracks through which the mechanical information can travel. By following the vectors of force created by the interactions of gravity, ground reaction force, momentum, and the joint alignment, we can easily see the contribution of the myofascial meridians to elastic efficiency, propulsion, stability, and shock absorption.

The multifaceted, three-dimensional fascial tissue of the Anatomy Trains uses shock absorption to stiffen the appropriate tissue in the vector of force on contact with the ground, and then it uses that stored energy to assist with propulsion in the opposite direction. In order to fully appreciate this, we must first analyze the activity at each of the joints during the gait cycle.

Joint Movement—Real and Relative

Working through the sequence of adaptations of the bones and joints will provide a consistent base of knowledge from which we can interpret the effects on the soft tissue. We will start with the foot and the most common place of first interaction with the walking surface, the heel. There are two ways in which we can analyze the movement of the skeletal system: the *real movement* of the bones and the *relative movement* at the joints. For example, the tibia rotates medially after heel strike, and this encourages the femur to rotate inward as well. However, the amount of inward rotation of the two bones is not necessarily the same, which creates a relative movement within the joint. If the tibia has moved farther and faster than the femur, we would describe the tibia as being medially rotated at the knee joint. The action at the joint will be determined by the *relative motion,* the amount by which one bone has moved in relation to the other. However, if the femur somehow medially rotated farther and/or faster than the tibia, it would create a relative external rotation at the joint (see fig. 2.7).

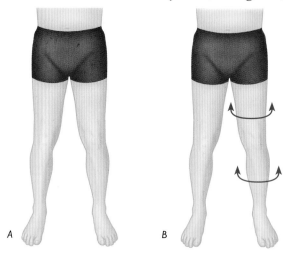

A   B

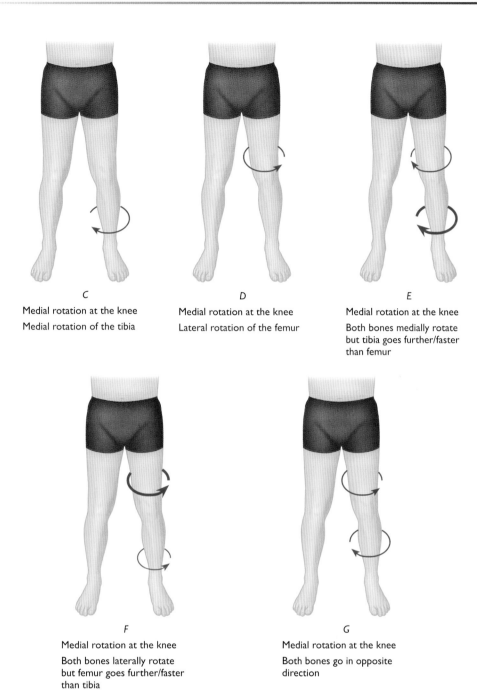

C
Medial rotation at the knee
Medial rotation of the tibia

D
Medial rotation at the knee
Lateral rotation of the femur

E
Medial rotation at the knee
Both bones medially rotate
but tibia goes further/faster
than femur

F
Medial rotation at the knee
Both bones laterally rotate
but femur goes further/faster
than tibia

G
Medial rotation at the knee
Both bones go in opposite
direction

Figure 2.7. If we start with the two lower limb bones in neutral (A), we have six options for movement. If they both move in the same direction and at the same real speed (B), there is no relative change or motion at the joint. To create a relative medial rotation at the knee joint, we either medially rotate the tibia (C) or laterally rotate the femur (D). If both bones move, we can get the same relationship across the joint by the tibia rotating farther and/or faster than the femur (E). If the femur moves farther/faster, relative medial rotation is created at the knee (F), even though the real motion is in the same direction as in E. If both bones go in opposite directions (G), the relative motion will be defined by the direction in which the distal bone moved. Note: the relationship at the joint is defined by the position of the distal bone in the body except when referring to the spine, where it is the superior bone that defines the relationship.

These two methods of analyzing the movements of the skeletal system are also called *arthrokinematic* (joint centered, with the two bones moving relative to each other) or an *osteokinematic* (bone centered and "real," that is, the actual movement of the bones in space). To fully describe the events of gait, we will, at times, need to use both conventions to appreciate what is happening in the soft tissue.

The Adaptation of the Foot

The first contact of the foot with the ground is perhaps the most important event in this chain. It is the first stage of "stance" phase (see table above), and it will define what happens throughout the rest of the body, provided the body can accept and adapt to this impact: tensegrity in action.

The ankle complex is only the first in a series of joints that should absorb some of the shock of impact. The knee and then the hip will be the next major shock absorbers, followed by the spine. It is, therefore, the accumulation of small corrections that both spread the load of the shock and also stimulate the appropriate myofascial response.

With the foot in front of the body and the first contact coming to the heel, the ground reaction force will be angled posteriorly and superiorly, causing the ankle to plantarflex and decelerate (see fig. 2.8).

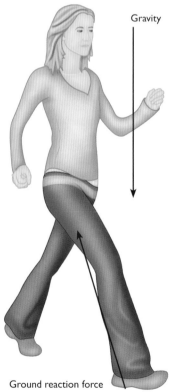

Gravity

Ground reaction force

Figure 2.8. Impact with the ground leads to a quick deceleration of the foot of the swing leg, and the interaction of the forward momentum of the foot and the ground reaction force will create a strong deceleration of the calcaneus.

Some writers have described the form of the back of the foot as a flawed design, due to the greater portion of body weight being transferred through the talus, which is not fully on top of the calcaneus (see fig. 2.9). This design, however, is essential for the easy, economical, and shock-absorbing walking that we all aim for. On a firm surface, the calcaneus will be brought to an abrupt stop, but the body's momentum will still be bearing down on top of it. A significant portion of the weight coming onto it is resting on a ledge of bone known as the sustentaculum talus—sometimes referred to as the "waiter's tray"—and this arrangement creates the ability for the calcaneus to tilt under the weight descending through the talus (see fig. 2.9).

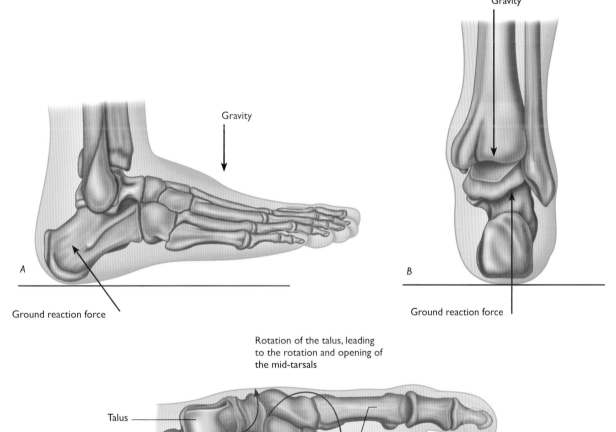

Figure 2.9. At heel strike, the position of the calcaneus will act like one end of a see-saw and force the foot into a sudden plantarflexion (A), medially tilt the calcaneus, also referred to as "eversion" (B), and, finally, medially rotate the calcaneus—and therefore the talus and lower limb—as the talus slides down the offset sustentaculum talus (C).

The eversion of the calcaneus (approximately 5 degrees) causes the talus to also tilt medially and to rotate medially. This movement within the subtalar joint affects the joints between the talus and both the navicular and the cuboid. Because of this, the more proximal tarsal bones will rotate more quickly, which will create a relative lateral rotation in the foot's distal joints (see fig. 2.10). This movement of the metatarsal bones of the foot affords them more freedom to adapt to the potentially random ground surface. This relaxation of the "form closure" (the natural support of the structure via its boney structure in a similar fashion to the "closure" given to a stone archway due to the shape of the blocks) of the foot also assists in sending the shock to the thick plantar tissues, spreading the force more widely.

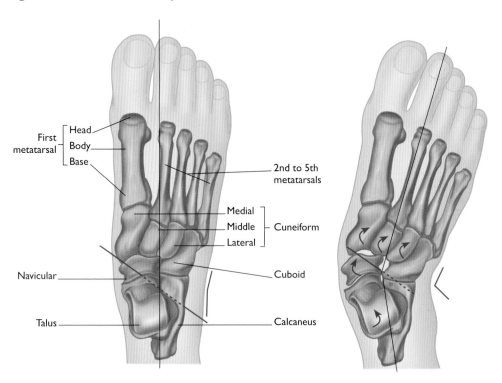

Figure 2.10. Following heel strike, the calcaneus and talus will very quickly rotate medially. The navicular and cuboid follow more slowly and therefore create a relative lateral rotation at their joints with the talus. This unlocks the midtarsal joint and allows the midtarsals to open and adapt to the ground.

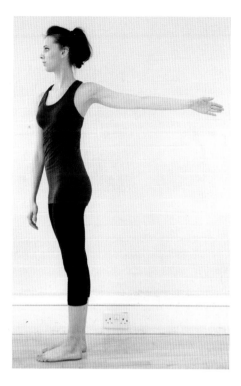

Figure 2.11. Feeling the movement of the midtarsal bones in exercise 2.1.

Exercise 2.1. To feel the opening of the bones of the foot, stand with both feet quite close together and parallel. Bring one or both hands in front of you and turn as far as comfortable to your left (as shown above), keeping both feet on the ground. Be sure to allow your pelvis to move with you. Try to move the midtarsal bones within the right foot. Compare that sensation to the movement available on the left. You should feel more movement on the right, because the heel of that foot is more internally rotated, similar to the action at heel strike.

The Adaptation of the Leg

The eversion of the calcaneus causes a medial rotation of the talus, which, in turn, causes a medial rotation of the tibia and fibula, since the talus is held in a mortise-and-tenon joint by the two leg bones (see fig. 2.12). The tibia and fibula medially rotate approximately 4 to 8 degrees as the knee flexes and comes across the front of the body, producing a valgus relationship at the knee joint (*valgus* refers to the angle created between the two bones forming the knee. In a valgus position, the tibia will angle down and out away from the femur).

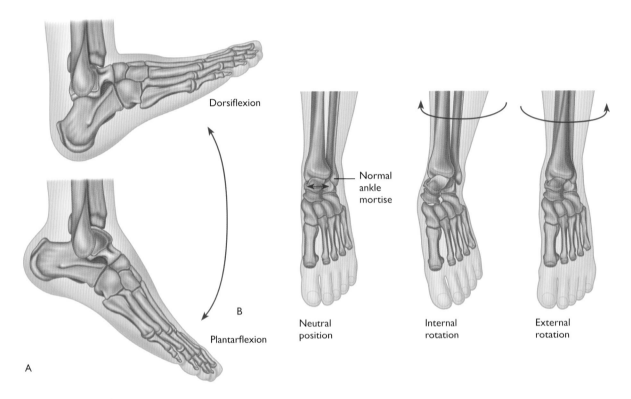

Figure 2.12. *The mortise-and-tenon arrangement of the bones of the talar joint allows an independent motion of the foot in the sagittal plane of motion—plantarflexion and dorsiflexion (A). When a transverse motion is introduced, the three bones will follow each other, because of the security inherent in this type of joint (B). This is the cause of the difference of movement in the two feet in exercise 2.1. If you try the exercise again, you will sense that your right and left legs are internally and externally rotated, respectively. The rotation of the lower leg affects the positioning of the talus. This will be important for the reversal of the joint relationship via the Deep Front Line later in the gait cycle (see chapter 6).*

The medial rotation of the tibia will draw the femur into a medial rotation as well, and the femur's rotation—along with the reach of the step—will cause the pelvis to rotate in the same direction.

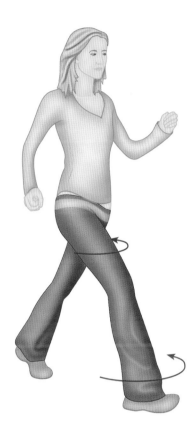

Figure 2.13. As we progress up the leg, all of the bones are moving in the same direction (osteokinematics) and the relationship at the joints (arthrokinematics) is a medial rotation: the bones are all moving medially, but, because of the different speeds and degrees of movement, the inferior bone at each joint is medially rotated when compared to its superior neighbor.

At the knee, the tibia and femur are both medially rotating, but the tibia is moving faster and farther than the femur. This means that the relative relationship between the two bones will be a medial rotation (of the tibia compared to the femur) at the knee. In the hip joint, the femur and pelvis are rotating in the same direction—medially—but the pelvis will have rotated away from the swing leg during the stride, and, therefore, the joint will be laterally rotated. This lateral rotation is increased, because the need for distance in the step causes more rotation of the pelvis, which pivots around the weight-bearing femur (see chapter 3).

Weight Acceptance

After heel strike, as the weight is transferred to the lower limb, the knee will flex from its relatively straight angle at heel strike (by anything up to 20 degrees), and the hip will adduct (by approximately 4 to 5 degrees) as the pelvis receives the weight of the upper body (see fig. 2.14).

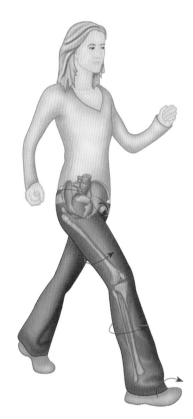

Figure 2.14. As the weight is passed to the forward limb, the knee flexes for additional shock absorption. Because the body's center of gravity is medial to the hip joint, the pelvis is encouraged into adduction as the laterally facing hip abductors receive the weight of the upper body and contract to keep it upright. This tilt of the pelvis has to be corrected in the spine before reaching the head—much of this is achieved by the lower three lumbar vertebrae.

While most of the lateral tilt of the pelvis is lessened by the adaptation of the lumbars (detailed in chapter 4), the lumbars are much less able to reduce the rotation of the pelvis. The body has a number of mechanisms to contain rotation, the main one being the forward swing of the upper girdle on the opposite side, which helps rotate the upper thoracics in opposite direction of the rotation of the pelvis. The rotation coming up from the pelvis and lower limbs therefore "meets" the counterrotation of the upper thoracics, and they cancel each other out before the movement reaches the neck and head (detailed in chapter 5).

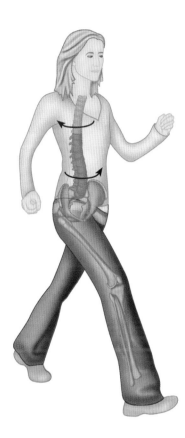

Figure 2.15. As the right foot heel strikes, the pelvis will be rotated to the left, which will also rotate the sacrum and the lumbars to the left. This is partly counterbalanced by the swing of the arms in the opposite direction, encouraging the upper thoracics to rotate to the right. These two rotational forces should balance each other out somewhere around T8.

All of the above actions occur at heel strike, as the foot receives the weight of the upper body. The deceleration of the foot as it contacts the ground causes a roll on the calcaneus, plantarflexing the foot. The foot, now firmly planted, cannot move farther forward (unless walking on ice), so the momentum of the body forces the tibia and fibula to pivot in the talar joint, similar to a vaulter's pole, which, when one end is brought to the ground, pivots to lift the other end. The pivot of the tibia and fibula brings the foot through into dorsiflexion until the posterior tissues at the ankle reach the limit of their range of motion. At that point, the additional forward motion of the body will cause the foot to roll onto the ball of the foot (see fig. 2.16, overleaf).

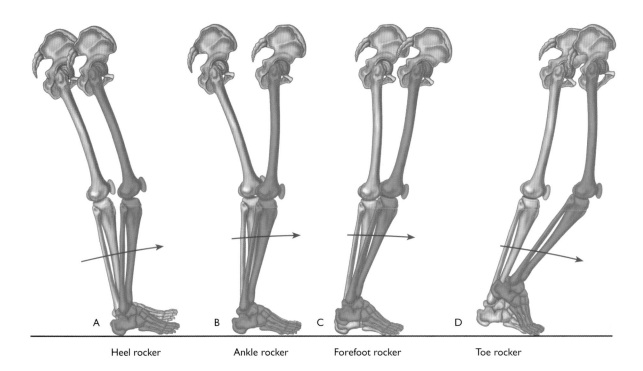

| Heel rocker | Ankle rocker | Forefoot rocker | Toe rocker |

Figure 2.16. The four stages that lead to the push-off for forward propulsion. The initial heel strike (A) and receiving of body weight cause the foot to brake, come into plantarflexion, and have full contact with the ground. This process causes the midtarsal joints to open and allows the foot to adapt with a slightly lowered arch, which also spreads the force of the impact to deeper tissues beyond the plantar fascia. The swing of the opposite leg (B) and progress of the pelvis and trunk, will cause the tibia and fibula to dorsiflex over the foot and then the heel to lift, creating a rocking motion on the ball of the foot (C), leading to the push-off from the ends of the metatarsals and the toes (D).

The swing of the opposite leg is what leads to the correction of the rotations that occurred from heel strike. As the swing leg comes through from posterior to anterior, it will, by necessity, turn the pelvis in the opposite direction. The movement of the pelvis will then laterally rotate the femur of the planted leg, which will rotate the tibia and fibula, and they will finally rotate the talus and, therefore, the calcaneus.

This brings us back to exercise 2.1. The bones of the medially rotating foot are in a loose and adaptable form, while those of the laterally rotated foot are much more solid and stable. It is important to remember we need this correction back to an integrated, stable foot to prepare for push-off. The loose foot, ideal for molding to the impact surface, becomes a more solid foot for rolling forward onto the ball of the foot prior to push-off (see fig. 2.17).

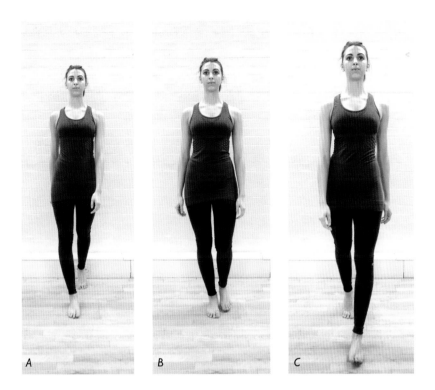

Figure 2.17. The rotation is determined by what is moving fastest at any one time. At the moment of heel strike, it is the eversion of the calcaneus that determines the chain of events upward into the rest of the body, as described above. Once the forward foot is planted on the ground (A), the back leg will then be accelerating from its push-off, and its momentum and anterior reach will turn the pelvis to the opposite side, creating a correcting rotation through the forward leg (B and C).

The Rest of the Body

The upper body will also continuously adapt through the gait cycle. The movement and angulation of the pelvis and the swing of the arms are two of the keys for understanding the body's movement. Any movement created in the lower body will have to be diminished before it reaches the head, in order for the eyes to remain steady and for the brain not to be traumatized by heel strike. The three-dimensional movement through the spine will be best explained through the discussion of the Anatomy Trains later, particularly in chapters 3 through 5.

The arms are especially used to counterbalance the forces going to the head in each of the planes of movement, but they also contribute to the elastic forces acting through the trunk, especially in oblique planes, and each arm works with the movement of the leg on the opposite side. While the upper body makes a significant contribution to walking, its actions are somewhat more straightforward and will be discussed later, in the context of the Anatomy Train lines.

THE SEQUENCE OF EVENTS AND THE SOFT TISSUE RESPONSE

The main focus of the next few chapters will be an analysis of the positions of the body at the two extremes: heel strike (including the process of weight acceptance) and push-off. It is at these points that the soft tissue is most engaged, stretched across the joints, and carrying more force, as the point of contact with the ground will be farther form the body's center of gravity.

At heel strike and push-off, the tissue is preparing for the naturally determined corrections throughout the rest of the body. By first understanding the pattern created in the bones and joints, we can look at where the force of impact is directed to in the soft tissues. We can see how the skeletal mechanics are detected by the proprioceptive system in the myofascia, which alert the appropriate muscles to decelerate downward movement of the body caused by the interaction of momentum, gravity, and ground reaction force. With this mechanism of deceleration in place, the body can reverse the sequencing of the chain with maximum efficiency, by using all of the elements of the stretch shortening cycle and fascial recoil that allow walking to be energy efficient, easy, and graceful.

At heel strike, the impact of the calcaneus initiates a sequence of events, a cascade of pronation movements channeled by the joints into the soft tissue. It unlocks the midtarsal joints and medially rotates the lower limb. The leg's medial rotation soon changes into a lateral rotation, caused by the swing of the opposite leg, transmitted through the pelvis. The lateral rotation of the tibia and fibula then encourages the supination of the foot via those bones' "clamping" of the talus. This supination realigns the midtarsal joints and force closes the joints of the foot, creating a stronger support for push-off.

It is the folding of the joints that creates the prestress—the countermovement or preparatory movement—that stimulates the muscle spindles to initiate an isometric contraction. That tightening of the muscles allows the associated fascia to absorb any further deceleration force. Once the fascia is at its elastic transition point, it can recoil like a spring. Furthermore, any requisite concentric contraction of the muscle is made more powerful as it pushes against the taut surrounding bag of tissues—the combined epimysium, endomysium, and perimysium.

If there is a fault in this system—if one joint movement is missing—muscle fibers somewhere along the chain may not be switched on, causing others to compensate. We recognize the fault when we feel we must make a special effort to continue moving. The next chapters will trace in more detail the important events in the joints that enhance the tissues' abilities to function with elastic kinetic energy along the Anatomy Train Lines.

3 Superficial Front and Superficial Back Lines

Walking: the most ancient exercise and still the best modern exercise.
—Carrie Latet

INTRODUCTION

Flexion and extension are probably the most obvious movements we see in walking, and they have generally been the focus of most analysis. Recently, in some fields of bodywork, it has become almost trendy to talk only about the rotational aspect of walking, but, as we will see, gait is truly a combination of all three planes, each of equal importance and interdependence.

When we look below the hip, the predominant joint alignment we see is in the sagittal plane, dealing with the movements of flexion and extension. That is not to say important elements of frontal and transverse planes are not present, but they will be dealt with in chapters 4 (Lateral Line) and 5 (Spiral Line), respectively. To better understand the strategies invoked by the body to offset the pull of gravity and to ensure easy, fluid movement, we will also need to look at the Functional Lines and the Deep Front Line. While some of the tissues of these lines overlap, they each give an extra support or add an essential vector to help correct or prepare for movement at different phases. But that will have to wait for later chapters. This chapter will concentrate on sagittal plane mechanics, and we will see how the bipedal gait naturally creates rotation by striding with one leg in front of the other.

A SERIES OF CONTROLLED FALLS

With each step, we have to stop ourselves from falling. When the foot hits the ground, significant downward force is absorbed by the body's soft tissues, and much of that work is done by the hip and knee extensors, which act against gravity to prevent additional flexion. As we saw in chapter 1, it is this folding of the joints—an inherent instability in the system—that provides shock absorption (i.e., it protects the brain from jiggling around) and provides metabolically cheap elastic energy. The downward motion loads the springs within the myofascia (see fig. 3.1).

As the swing leg progresses past the rockers of the planted foot, a gentle rise of the body is created, as the body rises onto the forefoot of the planted foot. The body sinks again at heel strike. This upward and downward movement appears to assist much of the loading of the elastic tissues to take advantage of the stretch shortening cycle. The rise of the body is necessary to create the potential energy that turns to kinetic (i.e., moving) energy on the fall, and the deceleration of this momentum is what feeds the stretch of the elastic tissues to provide the elastic recoil.

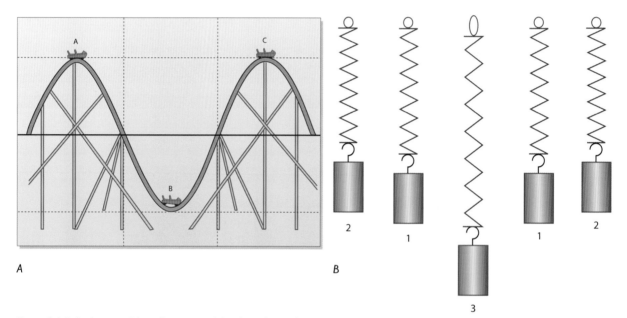

Figure 3.1.A, As the car of the roller coaster glides down the track it builds the kinetic energy that is used to ascend the next rise. At the top, much of the kinetic energy has been used up (as work), but, because of its new position on the apex of the ride, the car now has a lot of potential energy. This potential energy quickly becomes kinetic, once the car is on the downward side of the rise and starts to accelerate. B, The downward motion of the weight is decelerated by the resistance of the spring. This means that the kinetic energy of the downward movement is transferred into the spring, which reaches a point at which the force applied by the weight is matched by the elastic strength of the spring, and no more downward movement occurs. This is the same point as the roller coaster being at the top of the rise—we now have enough potential energy stored in the spring to "bounce" the weight back up.

A study by Ortega and Farley showed that reducing vertical displacement of the head (i.e., the up/down "bounce" of walking) led to an increase in metabolic work—the muscles had to work harder (2005). This seems contradictory to traditional thinking, which would suggest minimalizing up/down movement would be more energy efficient. However, momentum is needed by the body to create the pre-stretch in the elastic tissue that is part of our bipedal efficiency. That momentum is provided both by gravity and by the body's forward movement, utilizing the elastic characteristics of the front and back lines.

Much research has focused on the up/down movement of the body and less has considered the effects of loading the sagittal plane tissue, other than as individual muscle units. This chapter demonstrates that we can combine the use of gravity with forward movement to create effective loading of tissue in the Superficial Front and Superficial Back Lines.

GETTING STARTED—ONCE WITH GRAVITY

The longest journey begins with a single step.
—Lao Tsu

The benefits gained from preloading may be one reason why we pass our body weight on to our swing leg before we begin walking. When standing and intending to take a step, our body weight shifts briefly (and unconsciously) from being centrally placed between the feet toward the leg to be lifted, before transferring across to the weight-bearing side (see fig. 3.2). This suggests that vertically loading the swing leg may assist with recoiling it up and forward.

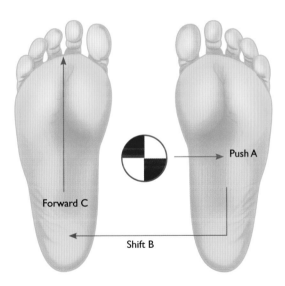

Figure 3.2. Pressure plate analysis shows that, in preparation for the first step, we move our center of gravity onto the swing leg momentarily before bringing it onto the stance side to initiate the step. This may help to mechanically load the tissue of the swing leg to assist with lifting and propelling it forward. By bringing the body weight onto the swing leg, the tissues will be loaded and potentially deformed a little to provide a spring to assist its first lift (adapted from Perry and Burnfield 2010).

Vertical displacement is related to body size and speed, and if we increase speed, we also increase vertical movement, giving us more downward momentum to stretch and load the elastic tissues to provide kinetic energy on their release. This change in strategy may explain some alterations we see in gait as speed increases. This was noticed by Hoyt and Taylor, who measured the energy costs of different speeds for ponies (in Vogel 2001). They found that the animals chose the particular speed for each gait—walk, trot, or gallop—that was the most energy efficient, that is, the different styles of movement led to optimum elastic loading.

You can feel this for yourself by going for a walk and gradually speeding up. When you are going fast enough, you will naturally switch to a jog and then to a run and eventually to a sprint. After each change, you can feel that you regain some efficiency, as the progression allows you to take advantage of the stretch shortening cycle, with reduced muscle effort. It is important to remember, however, that many factors will be involved in this, including speed, muscle strength, and biomechanics. This book predominately traces the most efficient and common biomechanical paths that take advantage of the myofascial chains.

The Superficial Front and Back Lines (SFL and SBL) have portions of their lines engaged via the upward/downward movement of the body at different times in the gait cycle, and they come into full engagement at either end—heel strike and push-off—when the tissues across the joints are required to lengthen (see figs. 3.3 and 3.4). Chapter 2 described how the full engagement of the joints allows transfer of force across the joints, from one body section to another.

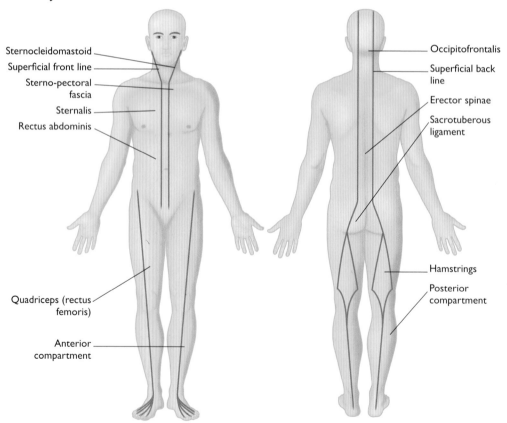

Figure 3.3. The Superficial Front and Back Lines make a significant contributions to the gait cycle. To take full advantage of their elastic recoil, they must be under stretch at push-off and heel strike.

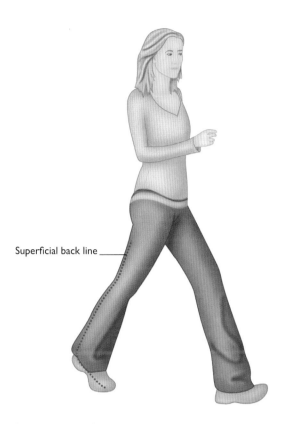

Superficial back line _____

Figure 3.4. The Superficial Back Line also makes a significant contribution to the gait cycle. To take full advantage of its elastic recoil, it needs to be under stretch at heel strike.

It is when most of the line is stretched, usually when one foot is behind or in front of both the pelvis and rib cage, that the myofascia can transfer the vertical force of gravity into forward or backward momentum (i.e., when the hip is flexed or extended). The continuities can be seen as the "containing springs" for the body that perceive instability in any direction and stiffen to maintain stability, and that then transfer the forces from kinetic to elastic in the opposite direction. We will explore this concept further in the Deep Front and Spiral Lines, in our discussion of Zorn and Hodeck's "Swingwalker" model.

PUSH-OFF

The SFL is tensioned by the leg being brought into hip and knee extension at the point of pushing off, and it uses that stored energy to assist with the swing phase, bringing the limb into flexion in preparation for heel strike. At that point the predominant tension reverts to the SBL, as the back of the body has to contract strongly to resist gravity.

As the pelvis moves forward over the planted foot, the fascia of the SFL will be passively tensioned by the momentum of the skeleton (see fig. 3.5, overleaf). The hip joint and the lumbars come into extension, lengthening the rectus femoris and rectus abdominis, along with their associated fascia. This will contribute some fascial recoil for the flexion that will be required for the next swing phase, once the stage of push-off is achieved again.

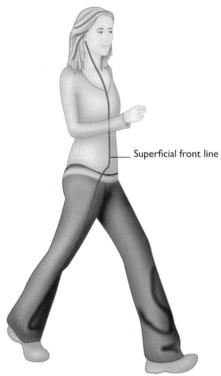

Superficial front line

Figure 3.5. The progression of the skeleton moving over the foot creates a natural tension within most of the Superficial Front Line.

GETTING STARTED—A SECOND TIME WITH SAGITTAL LOADING

Dalton, Bishop, Tillman, and Haas demonstrated that placing the swing foot slightly behind the stance foot prior to taking the first step can increase forward propulsion and decrease the amount of time required for starting the step (2011). This was found to be effective if the swing foot is placed only half a foot behind the stance foot, which pre-tensions both the hip flexors and the foot plantarflexors. This simple repositioning was successful for both older adults and for those diagnosed with Parkinson's disease, and it can be easily explained by the pre-tensioning of the tissue within the SFL as well as the lower portion of the SBL.

Exercise 3.1. One can quite easily feel the positive effect of the SFL tensioning by tapping your toe on the floor behind you. Try this by reaching back quite quickly with one foot to touch the floor behind you and then relaxing, trying not to actively bring your leg back to its starting position. It will come back of its own volition, using the energy that has been put into the tissue of the Superficial Front Line by the

posterior swing of the leg stretching its elastic elements. You may need to experiment a little before really getting the sense of it, but try at various speeds and with different amounts of force, and also try increasing the amount of time you allow the toe to stay on the floor behind you. Most people feel that increasing the speed increases the recoil, as does a longer range of motion, but only as far as you can go before the other hip has to flex, which compromises the continuity of the Superficial Front Line. Timing is also crucial—spend too long with your toe on the floor behind you, and you lose the momentum. This is the *amortization effect:* too long a pause, and much of the elastic loading is lost, wasted as heat and causing an increase in active work to return the leg forward again.

Exercise 3.1 gives us a possible explanation of why the Dalton experiment found a positive result from displacing the swing foot. Even a slight pre-tension within the tissue will lessen the amount of muscle work and coordination necessary to begin the leg swing. The leg extension has provided elastic potential energy that can be used for the returning flexion.[1]

Preloading a tissue removes any slack from the fascial elements—it "shrink wraps" the fascia around the muscle—which means that once the muscles contained within the fascia are required to contract, the force created by the muscles is immediately transferred through the fascia's length. This effectively reduces the work required of the muscles and increases their relative power.

The Superficial Front Line may also give us food for thought on the implications of structural and functional positioning of the upper body while walking. Try repeating exercise 3.1 with an anterior head position, with your rib cage in various tilts or shifts, and with your arms and shoulders in protraction and retraction. Each of these will influence the amount of "spring" you feel in the hip and so may need to be addressed in a client with compromised gait efficiency (see Clinical Note below).

Clinical Note

Is the tensioning of the SFL part of the reason for your client's posterior tilt of the rib cage? If the head is held in an anterior position, it can shorten the SFL (see fig. 3.6A), and the posterior tilt of the thorax is a common compensation (see fig. 3.6B). The posterior tilt of the thorax predominately acts as a counterbalance to the acquired head position, but it may also assist with the tension created at the front to help the recoil into flexion during gait.

---

1 It is called 'potential' energy because it has not yet been used; it can be converted into other events. In the case of elastic energy, the potential produced is generally for movement in the opposite direction.

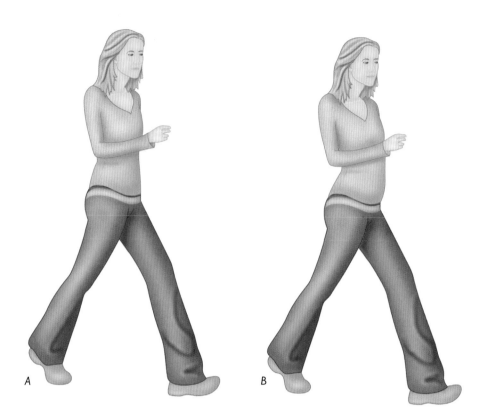

Figure 3.6. With an anteriorly shifted head, the fascia of the SFL may not be as effectively tensioned by hip extension (A), and this may be compensated for by posteriorly tilting the rib cage (B). In this way, both the SFL and the SBL will develop areas of restriction as the body tries to create a certain kind of balance.

Pre-swing

As the pelvis progresses over the foot, the knee begins to bend in the pre-swing phase, pushing out against the fascia of the SFL (see fig. 3.7). This further stimulates the connective tissue and could stimulate the muscles of the anterior compartment to contract in anticipation of lifting the foot and supporting it through the swing cycle. The extra fascial tension in the tibialis anterior may also have a role in the inversion/ supination of the medial arch, bringing it out of the eversion/inversion pattern created at heel strike, though it's more likely that there are stronger forces at work in that supination, as will be discussed later.

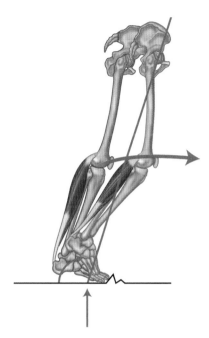

Figure 3.7. When the knee comes forward to prepare for the leg swing, it will push into the fascial line of the SFL (A), assisting with the lift of the leg and creating the signal for the muscles of the anterior compartment to begin contracting to lift and support the foot. EMG readings show the tibialis anterior and the long extensors all beginning to contract during the pre-swing phase and staying active until the weight is fully received by the foot in loading response (after Perry and Burnfield 2010).

Heel Strike and …

Just as the Superficial Front Line assists the recoil for flexion, the Superficial Back Line helps with extension. At heel strike, the foot is in front of the center of gravity and the hip is flexed, creating a lot of downward force behind the body's point of contact with the ground (see fig. 3.7). There are a number of fascial mechanisms that are automatically engaged in this position, the first of which is the SBL. With the hip flexed, the sacroiliac joint nutated, the knee extended, and the ankle dorsiflexed, the fascia of the SBL will be lengthened prior to heel strike. (As will be discussed later, the Lateral, Spiral, and Back Functional Lines also make a strong contribution to resisting gravity's desire for hip flexion, and by decelerating it, they encourage the forward propulsion into hip extension.)

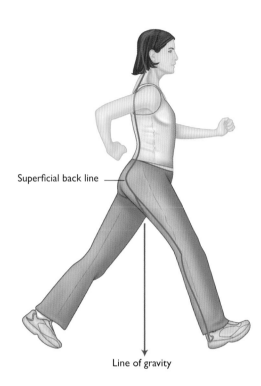

Superficial back line

Line of gravity

Figure 3.8. In the above position, the fascia of the Superficial Back Line is tensioned by the flexion at the hip (A). This appears to stimulate the supporting muscles of the hamstrings from mid-swing through to loading response, when the body is much more aligned over the foot (B). The initiation of contraction during mid-swing contributes to deceleration and control of the limb, but it also pre-tenses the myofascia to prepare for the stretch shortening cycle, taking advantage of the recoil to assist muscle contraction.

After being strongly loaded during heel strike, the SBL now has to lengthen in the lower section, below the knee, as the ankle moves into dorsiflexion. Ankle dorsiflexion will lengthen all of the plantarflexors, including those associated with the Lateral Line (the fibularii) and the Deep Front Line (the tibialis posterior and the flexors hallucis and digitorum longus). As they come forward to their natural end of range, they will decelerate the tibia, while the femur progresses more quickly above, bringing the knee joint into extension.

FOOT ROCKERS AND THE WINDLASS EFFECT

Walking is good for solving problems – it's like the feet are little psychiatrists.
—Pepper Giardino

Once the heel comes in contact with the floor, the ground reaction force, interacting with gravity and with momentum from the body, causes the foot to roll on the calcaneus (see fig. 3.9). This alteration of forces is similar to that of a pole vaulter planting the pole and changing the downward movement of the pole into forward and upward movement. The interaction of the calcaneus and the ground forms a braking mechanism, encouraging the "pole" of the leg to pass above it.

As the pelvis progresses over the planted foot, the ankle joint changes from being plantarflexed to dorsiflexed, and eventually it reaches the limit of its range, causing the heel to lift and the foot to rock onto the metatarsal heads and then quickly onto the toes.

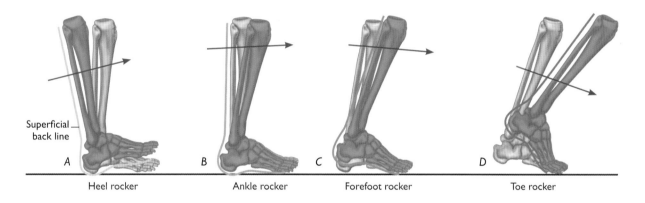

Figure 3.9. From heel strike, the rest of the limb "vaults" over the rocker of the calcaneus (A) and progresses into dorsiflexion via the talar joint, which tensions the SBL (B). As its natural range is met, the heel lifts to force the point of contact with the ground onto the rocker of the ball of the foot (C) and eventually onto the toes (D).

This creates four so-called rockers in the foot: the heel, ankle, forefoot, and toes. For smooth progression through each of these rockers, the joints must be free and the plantarflexors long enough to allow the full movement to occur. As we will see in the Deep Front Line and the Lateral Line, the tendons passing around the malleoli also have to be in balance to allow the foot to come back from the eversion/pronation created by heel strike and weight acceptance.

As the ankle rocker action lengthens the soleus and gastrocnemius (see fig. 3.10, overleaf), the foot will return to a neutral position by supinating and will reengage the midtarsal joints. This will allow the continuity of the soleus, gastrocnemius, and the plantar fascia to further support the many joints of the foot to give a smooth transition through the forefoot and toe rockers. If the mid-foot does not revert properly (i.e., if the midtarsal joints do not reengage into a locked position), undue stress may be placed on the plantar fascia, as it will be forced to become the main stabilizer of the foot.

Because the soleus, the deeper of the two calf muscles, attaches medially on the calcaneus, it also assists to draw the heel bone out of eversion. The soleus will have the cooperation of the Deep Front Line for this, due to the angle at which the tendons of the deep posterior compartment cross the subtalar joint (see chapter 6).

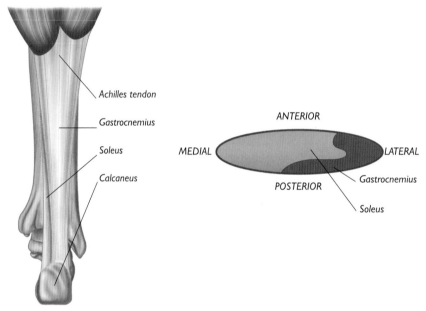

Figure 3.10. Due to its deeper and more medial attachment, the soleus can help bring the calcaneus into inversion, thereby helping the tarsal bones to realign. The gastrocnemius attachments are more lateral and superficial, with much of its fascial tissue being continuous around the heel and into the plantar fascia (see fig. 3.11). Adapted from Perry and Burnfield 2010.

The failure of any of the above "rockers" will prevent the foot from rolling through onto the toes for an effective push-off. The stride will naturally shorten and often a hip-hiking strategy, when the affected limb is "lifted" from the same side of the pelvis through to flexion, will be used in compensation. This compensation may appear regardless of the cause (it could be due to lack of hip extension, knee extension, ankle dorsiflexion, or loss of any of the foot rockers), and therefore some strategy must be developed for differential diagnosis to create a remedial plan.

Pulleys and the Windlass Effect

The dorsiflexion of the ankle is symbiotic with the inversion of the bones of the feet; both events assist the tensioning of the plantar tissue (see fig. 3.11). This gathering together of the bones of the foot and the tensioning of the elastic tissue creates the so-called windlass effect. The windlass is created by the plantarflexor tendons that wrap around the pulleys of the calcaneus and the malleoli; as the tibia moves over the foot into dorsiflexion, the lines of these tendons are drawn tight.

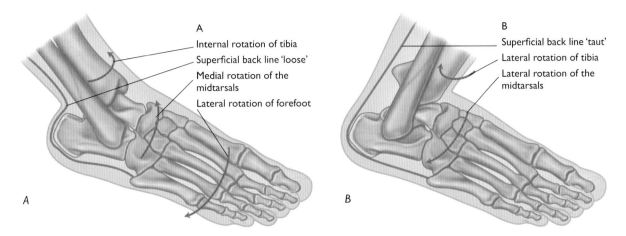

A
— Internal rotation of tibia
— Superficial back line 'loose'
— Medial rotation of the midtarsals
— Lateral rotation of forefoot

B
— Superficial back line 'taut'
— Lateral rotation of tibia
— Lateral rotation of the midtarsals

A

B

Figure 3.11. The plantar flexion at heel strike creates slack in the lower portion of the SBL, which allows the midtarsal joints and bones to open and adapt to the surface (A). Coming into dorsiflexion (B) tensions the soleus and gastrocnemius and thereby helps tension the plantar fascia, which draws the midtarsal bones back together and creates an integrated foot for push-off, the so-called windlass effect.

The eponymous tendon may have been Achilles's weak spot, but thankfully for the rest of us, it is one of the strongest areas in our bodies. The fibers from the soleus and gastrocnemius spiral by approximately 90 degrees into the tendon. This brings the soleus to the medial aspect of the calcaneus, where it can help produce inversion; it may also strengthen the calcaneus considerably (Doral et al. 2010). Despite its great strength, however, the Achilles tendon is still the third most ruptured tendon in the body—after the rotator cuff and the tendons of the knee—though this should not be surprising, when we consider that it has to handle forces up to twelve times our body weight.

The Achilles tendon, like the rest of the body, has been shown to be hugely adaptable, apparently increasing its cross-sectional area as usage increases. It has been found that the tendon in athletes in significantly thicker than in nonathletes. It should be noted, however, that the direction of the correlation is not fully established; it could be that a thicker Achilles tendon leads to better athletic performance (Malvankar and Khan 2011). Studies have also shown that there is a feedback between the stiffness of the tendon and the tension of the attaching/controlling muscles. The muscles will adjust their tension to match the elasticity of the tendon in order to maximize the efficiency of the elastic output (Lichtwark and Wilson 2007)—the further implications of this will be discussed in chapter 6.

The windlass effect is hugely dependent on the performance and strength of the Achilles tendon during push-off. The progression through to the toe rocker will tension the tendon, correcting the midtarsal joints and engaging the plantar fascia. The lengthening created by the progressive dorsiflexion will load the tissue significantly, creating a tremendous amount of energy that can be utilized to push the body forward when it is released.

This makes the Achilles tendon, along with the gluteus maximus, one of the most important anatomical factors for human gait. The human Achilles tendon is much longer than that of other primates—and the calf is less bulky—as the power is produced through elasticity rather than muscle contraction. This allows our lower leg to be lighter, which means that it takes less energy to move it. It also gives it the greatest velocity of any of our body parts, as well as the advantage of the larger tendon storage system assistance. We see this dynamic to a greater extent in the limbs of animals that use strong hip muscles to control long, slender, and tendinous hind limbs, such as horses, antelopes, and kangaroos.

Catapults

The effect of the foot rockers and the tensioning of the tissue that occurs through ankle dorsiflexion and knee extension creates a catapult mechanism. The forward momentum of the tibia and femur is decelerated by the isometric contraction of the plantarflexors. This leads to the mechanical loading of the elastic tissues, which are stretched until being finally released at push-off, once the foot has progressed over the toe rocker. The toes act as the final locking device, and once it is released, the stored energy in the elastic tissue can be released to assist with forward propulsion. This is triggered by full extension of the knee, which allows the hamstring and gastrocnemius tissue to link together as a continuous system, creating a smoother transfer of force from the proximal to distal bones of the leg.

Exercise 3.2

Much of the windlass effect is created within the lower leg, but one can feel the loss of power brought about by lack of knee extension by just taking a few steps without fully straightening the legs. Compare this to your normal gait (if you do bring the knee into extension!), and you feel how the engagement of the fascia across the knee joint greatly assists the power of the plantarflexion. Some of this may be explained by knee flexion shortening the gastrocnemius and therefore taking it out of the equation, but even a slight change in knee position makes more change than one would expect. This may be due to the interlocking effect of the fascia from the hamstrings, which more effectively engage with the plantarflexors when the knee is extended (see Myers 2009). With the knee not fully extended, some people may feel the increased range of motion as they come over to the toe rocker, losing the power of push-off. This is an example of how the integrity of the myofascial line can assist with a more effective transfer than single elements.

The catapult of the foot is assisted by a similar contrivance in the tissue that crosses the front of the hip with the Superficial Front Line. As the pelvis comes forward into hip extension, it will stretch the myofascia of the hip flexors. It can do this because of the "lock" created by the foot on the ground, which prevents the leg from coming forward too early. Once the foot progresses onto the toe rocker, the two catapults are released simultaneously—one for hip flexion and one for foot flexion. You may have felt the loss of this force in exercise 3.2, as the two work in concert, requiring the motion at the involved joints to be in balance in order to load and then release the springs effectively.

The spring of the SFL requires the release, or "trigger," mechanism of the toe rockers in order to propel the leg forward into flexion. Theoretically, without the release of the foot created from the toe rocker, the elastic tension created by the hip extension would encourage the pelvis backward rather than the leg forward.

Catapult mechanisms have been discussed in the movement of other animals, but little in that of humans. We follow similar strategies, albeit with less dramatic effects than the huge leaps of bush babies or the phenomenal shooting of curled lizard tongues. Being less specialized, our springs are of a more sedate nature but are nonetheless important contributors to the spring motions we gain from our elastic tissue.

The windlass and catapult reactions depend on a number of events—foot rockers all performing appropriately, as well as knee and hip extension—to bring the fascial lines into engagement, allowing the momentum of each body part to assist the movement of the others. Our range of motion is therefore crucial for graceful walking. Many experiments have been done comparing the efficiency of upright versus quadrupedal gait using trained chimpanzees. The design of the experiments was flawed from the start, because the chimps' joints have different ranges from ours and, therefore, will not allow the fascial engagement to occur.

Chimpanzees have a range of 45 degrees of dorsiflexion, which allows their feet to hold the trunk of a tree as they climb. This is far beyond the 20 degrees in humans. In order for the catapult or elastic mechanisms to work, we have to engage the fascial tissues in a stretch; a chimpanzee would need to be taking a very long stride to create enough dorsiflexion to pull on their Achilles tendon. Paleoanthropologists use ankle joints as an indicator of upright gait: by looking at the shape of the distal tibia, they can infer the joint's range of motion and the angle of transfer of force. In upright, bipedal gait, the body weight would be coming almost straight through the joint. In most quadrupeds, by contrast, it would be passing through the joint at an angle, as they remain more dorsiflexed as they move.

The first hominin fossil that we see with ankle joints that indicate a bipedal stance is "Lucy," possibly the world's most famous human ancestor, found by Donald Johanson in Ethiopia in 1974. Named after the Beatles' hit "Lucy in the Sky with Diamonds," Lucy has been confirmed as an example of *Australopithecus afarensis* and dates from approximately 3.2 million years ago. She was quite short, at around 3 feet, 7 inches, and her bones exhibit many features that show that Lucy walked consistently on two legs, including pelvic, femoral, and humeral changes (many other primates are only occasional bipeds). Lucy is the oldest fossil showing some of these changes in the leg bones. Many older fossils also show some signs of bipedalism, though their remains are not as complete as Lucy's, with few lower leg bones surviving in the fossil record so far.

If you revisit exercise 3.2, you may notice that not extending the knee coincided with decreased hip extension. This "bent-knee, bent-hip" gait is characteristic of nonhuman primates, but their use of the gait is due to their inability to create a lumbar lordosis rather than a lack of length in the tissue. What this means in terms of efficiency is that they cannot fully engage the long multi-joint fascial chains when walking upright, and thus they rely much more on muscle power.

Leg Springs

The lower leg has the greatest velocity of any of our body parts during walking and running. Minimizing its weight therefore has many benefits for energy conservation. By having longer, stronger tendons, the tendons can be used for greater energy storage, diminishing the need for heavy muscles in the calf. We see this arrangement frequently in the rest of the animal world, such as in horses, antelopes, and kangaroos, which use their strong hip muscles to control long, slender, and tendinous limbs (see fig. 3.12).

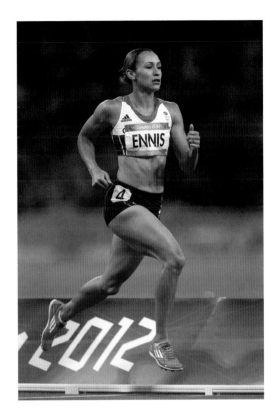
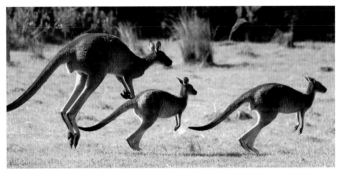
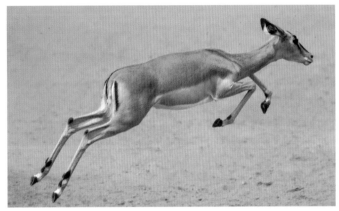

Figure 3.12. As in all elite runners, in comparison to the bulk of her upper body, Jessica Ennis's lower leg appears quite spindly. When compared to the elite "athletes" of the nonhuman animal kingdom, this arrangement of proximal muscles controlling the long, tendinous sections of the lower leg seems common. Jessica Ennis photograph courtesy of Getty Images. Kangaroo and antelope photographs courtesy of istock.com.

"Expresses" and "Locals"

Within his "Anatomy Trains" model, Myers discusses the concept of "expresses" versus "locals" (2009). He describes "local" muscles as those that cross one joint and "expresses" as those that cross two or more. We can use this concept to explain the catapult phenomenon. By allowing the hip and knee joints to extend and the ankle to dorsiflex, the "expresses" engage more fully across these areas with longer portions of the myofascial chains being put under stretch. Without the stretch, the tissue will have to actively contract to produce the required force for flexion.

The long chain stretches involved in an unrestricted stride therefore take the pressure off the deeper, usually "local" muscles. In the absence of elastic energy, the muscles will have to work and thereby potentially become overused. As other primates cannot extend their knees and hips, their muscles are highly developed compared to ours.

Pelvic Torsions (but in a Good Way)

During the swing of the leg forward toward heel strike, the fascia of the SBL on that leg is tensioned, which will contribute to the leg's ability to resist gravity once the calcaneus contacts the ground. Essentially, the flexion of the hip creates a pre-stretch of the hamstrings (as well as the other hip extensors, but we will concentrate on the tissue of the SBL for now) prior to heel strike. This preloads the elastic tissue and thereby enhances the power output of the antigravity muscles (the hamstrings, in this case), thus reducing the work they have to perform to prevent us falling to the ground.

As the leg swings through into hip flexion, the hamstrings will pull the ischial tuberosity with it, thereby encouraging the associated hip into a posterior tilt. On the other side, the hip will be going into extension, so the hip flexors will be tautening and pulling their hip into a relative anterior tilt.[2] The alternating and contralateral actions of the ilia create torsion within the pelvis, a movement that is allowed by the design of the sacroiliac joints at the back and the symphysis pubis at the front (see fig. 3.13).

Exercise 3.3. Place your hands on your iliac crests and walk. Can you feel the movement of the ilia under the tissue? Do you sense the ilia tilting back as you swing the leg forward and then tilting forward as the thigh extends? The SFL and SBL therefore seem to be involved in creating this torsion action through the pelvis (see fig. 3.13). This effect on the pelvis is an important driver of events for the Lateral and Spiral Lines (see chapters 4 and 5).

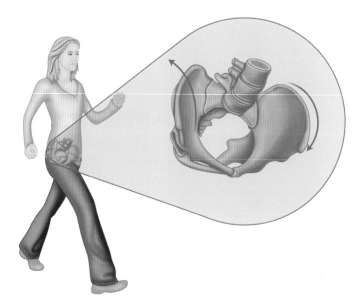

Figure 3.13. Bipedal gait puts many vectors of force through the pelvis, requiring it to adapt in all three planes of motion (sagittal, frontal, and transverse). The lengthening and shortening of the SFL and SBL on alternate sides creates tilting in the sagittal plane, which leads to the torsion in the pelvis.

2 We will revisit this in the Spiral Line, chapter 5, and discuss its significance for the sacroiliac joints.

The anterior tilt of the pelvis on the extended leg will tension—and thereby switch on—the abdominals on the same side. The ability of the pelvis to move is therefore essential to the functioning of the abdominals, and we will see later that the rotation and lateral tilt are necessary for the three dimensions of the "core" to be activated. The overall anterior tilt of the pelvis creates extension in the back and tensions the whole anterior aspect of the SFL to assist with hip flexion via the mechanical link of the pelvis, as outlined in Myers's Anatomy Trains (see fig. 3.14).

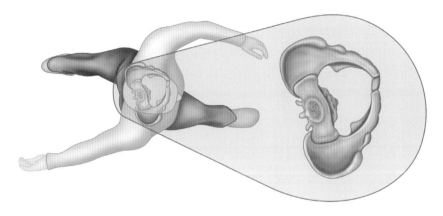

Figure 3.14. While walking, the pelvis is often in an overall anterior tilt (the posterior tilt of the ilium on the side of the flexed leg is relative to the resting tilt of the pelvis as a whole). As the leg extends, the pelvis acts as a mechanical link to connect the tensioning of the leg to the tissue of the upper SFL, engaging the fascial elasticity.

Exercise 3.4. Place one hand on your abdominals and go for a short walk. Can you feel the tissue over the rectus abdominis becoming taut as either leg goes into extension? Move your hand higher, to the sternum. Can you feel the strain in the tissue lying over the bone? Experiment with different speeds—do you feel more or less fascial tensioning as you increase your speed?

Rotation

Strangely, much of the rotation introduced to the body in walking, particularly to the pelvis, is initiated by the sagittal plane elements of the SFL and SBL. The forward swing of one leg will pull the hip on that side forward, via the hamstring attachment, and the opposite side will be held back by the tensioning of the SFL as the hip goes into extension. The combined effect, therefore, will be to rotate the pelvis, provided the stride is long enough to engage both lines. The contralateral forces of the opposing SFL and SBL are therefore essential for the creation of a series of events for the rest of the body, as well as for the engagement of many of the other lines.

When walking is observed from the side, there is an apparent 20-degree extension of the hip prior to push off. This is not pure extension, however, but rather an accumulation of events at different joints: the hip itself (which can extend up to 10 to 12 degrees), the anterior tilt of the connecting ilium (by between 3 and 7 degrees), and the backward rotation of the whole pelvis (between 8 and 12 degrees). The hip extension and anterior tilt of the ilium serve to assist with the preload of the SFL, SPL, and DFL (see chapters 5 and 6).

The rotation of the pelvis is required to help lengthen the stride. The pivoting action on the weight-bearing hip joint allows the opposite leg to reach farther forward. Experiment by walking with and without side-to-side pelvic rotation to feel the difference; to progress forward in the sagittal plane, the pelvis assists by rotating in the transverse plane.

The stride length, provided it is long enough, tensions the tissue of the SFL and SBL (along with other lines), but it also creates rotation in the pelvis (see fig. 3.15). Rotation of the pelvis rotates the sacrum, and the transverse motion is passed into the spine. As said earlier, we walk to take our heads and hands to other places. For our eyes to focus on our goal, our heads have to remain relatively steady, and so this rotation in the body has to be reduced before reaching the head.

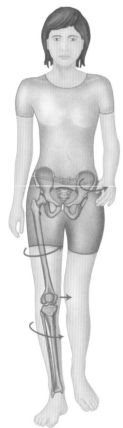

Figure 3.15. Our bipedal gait naturally causes us to rotate as we reach forward with alternate legs. This rotation at the pelvis is useful for the transfer of force into the Lateral and Spiral Lines, but it must be reduced before reaching the head.

Figure 3.16 shows the amount of rotation that is available at each spinal segment. Some of the rotation can be absorbed between L5/S1—the interface between the sacrum and the lowest lumbar—as it can rotate a few degrees, but the remaining rotational force will travel through the lumbars to reach the thoracics. The thoracic vertebrae have a much better range of motion in the transverse plane and are better able to reduce the rotation.

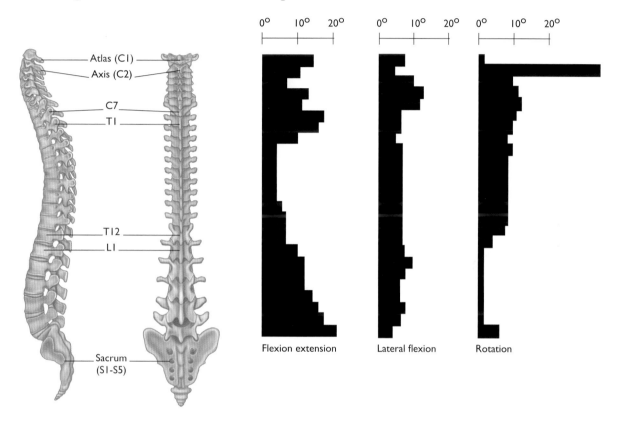

Figure 3.16. Each spinal segment varies in its abilities to move in each plane. The lumbar spine does not have much rotation ability, so this will send the pelvic rotation up to the thoracic vertebrae.

The facet joints of the lumbar vertebrae are predominately arranged in the sagittal plane, allowing for a wide range of flexion and extension—part of what allows us an upright, bipedal gait, as it gives us the ability to create lumbar lordosis (see fig. 3.17, overleaf). This arrangement restricts rotation, however, as the facets will encroach on one another in the transverse plane.

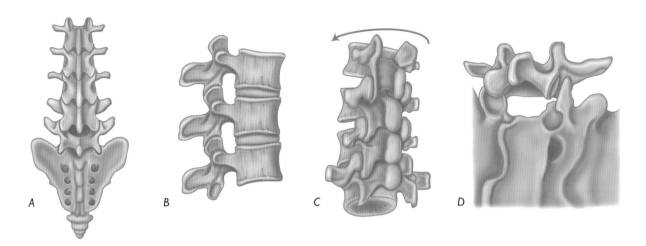

Figure 3.17. The vertical orientation of most of the lumbar facet joints (A) allows a great deal of flexion and extension (B) but limits rotation, as they quickly interface with each other (C). The exception to this is the joint at L5/S1, which, due to L5's need to grab on to the tilted sacrum, has facets that are turned a little more to the frontal plane and can therefore allow a little more rotation between the two surfaces (D).

As we will see in chapter 5, the limitation of the lumbar spine is very useful: by encouraging the rotation up to the thoracics, it allows the contralateral forces of the Spiral Line to meet and recoil.

ESSENTIAL EVENTS

Matching Triggers

At the point of push-off, two catapult mechanisms have been created, one for push-off and one for hip flexion, in the SBL and SFL, respectively. Ideally, both of these are discharged simultaneously, allowing the elastic energy of the lower SBL to produce plantarflexion and assisting the release of the SFL for hip flexion—each force encouraging the forward propulsion of the extended leg.

For that to happen, a number of sagittal plane events must take place. We need to roll through each of the foot rockers—heel, ankle, mid-foot, and toe—and the knee and the hip must extend. The lumbar and thoracic spine must also extend. Finally, the head should preferably be kept upright to engage the SFL and assist with flexion of the leg.

Heel Rocker

Our calcaneus is much larger than that of other primates, meaning that we have a larger contact surface to dissipate the force at heel strike. This function is assisted by the presence of a thick fat pad under the calcaneus (which absorbs approximately 17 percent to 19 percent of the impact force) and by the make-up of the bone itself, which is quite pliable. Any changes in either of these tissues, often caused by localized trauma, can cause a protective limp to develop. The stride will shorten to avoid or minimize heel strike, and the contact time of the affected foot with the ground will decrease.

The rounded aspect of the calcaneus should be able to comfortably make contact with the ground and, because of its position behind the talar joint, encourage the foot to plantarflex and interface with the surface. Any number of factors may influence its ability to perform its duty as the first point of contact—heel spurs and plantar fasciitis being the two most common.

Ankle Rocker

Immediately following heel strike, the ankle should plantarflex by approximately 10 degrees, a movement controlled and decelerated by the anterior compartment (the tibialis anterior, in particular). Failure of these muscles leads to foot slap and the lack of proper absorption of the force of impact. Loss of function in these muscles can often be due to neurological deficit (for example, a stroke or compartment syndrome–type compressions) and should therefore be managed by a physician.

The progression of the tibia and fibula over the talus can be restricted for a number of reasons. Apparent shortness of the posterior compartment (SBL) is the first and most obvious, but as we will see in future chapters, it can also be due to limits of the soft tissue of the deep posterior and lateral compartments, of the Deep Front Line and Lateral Line, respectively. Limits in these areas will also affect the transverse plane balance in the foot, due to their medial and lateral pathways around the ankle.

Because the talus is wider at the front of the bone than the back, the tibial and fibular malleoli must spread in order to accommodate it in dorsiflexion (see fig. 3.19). This mortise-and-tenon design means that when the foot is dorsiflexed, the talus is locked for extra ankle stability. The opening of the bones requires both the adaptability within the interosseous membrane between the two bones and also the ability of the fibula to move on the lateral aspect of the proximal tibia. While soft tissue manipulation and stretching may be effective in dealing with the limits in myofascial range, some form of bone manipulation may be required if the dorsiflexion is restricted by the joint interface. This can be due to congenital issues, if the talus is too wide or too flat at the front to interface correctly between the malleoli. In these cases, slight heel lifts may be a possible solution, which will provide relative dorsiflexion and reduce any compensation into pronation and medial push-off.

The differences in cause of the limits can be assessed using a simple knee bend or squat, as described below (see fig. 3.18*B*).

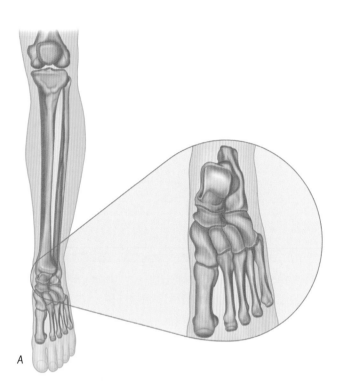

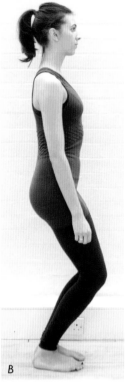

A

B

Figure 3.18. A, The tibia and fibula must be able to separate slightly on dorsiflexion to accommodate the greater width at the front of the talus. Limitations can develop within the interosseous membrane or at the proximal tibio-fibular joint, but these can often be manipulated to improve range. Bony changes at the front of the talus may also occur, either acquired or present from birth, creating permanent restriction. B, When the client squats to the end of range in dorsiflexion, he or she may feel a "block" either behind the ankle (usually indicating a soft tissue issue) or at the front (which is likely to indicate a joint restriction).

The less common issue of too much dorsiflexion may lead to overuse strains on the posterior myofascia and is only an issue during high or increased usage.

Mid-Foot Rocker

Prior to push-off, body weight should ideally progress onto the first and second metatarsal heads. The first metatarsal is wider and stronger than any of the other toes and is clearly designed to carry more force through it, but in order to create a stable push-off, its length needs to be relatively matched to that of the second metatarsal.

In the 1920s, physician and evolutionary anatomist Dudley J. Morton discovered that approximately 15 percent of the population has what came to be known as "Morton's Foot." In this condition, the second metatarsal is more than 8 millimeters longer than the first, and when the foot progresses toward push-off, it will be doing so on a single point rather than two. This encourages the foot to "fall" to one side or the other, leading into a rotation (see fig. 3.19). If the metatarsals are of significantly different lengths, an orthotic correction (a Morton's extension) may be necessary.

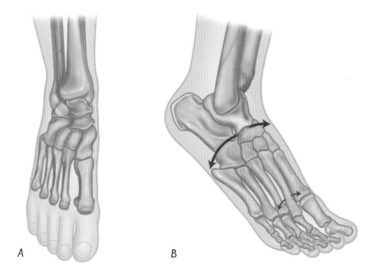

A   B

Figure 3.19. Ideally, the first and second metatarsals will be of equal length (A), which will create a stable platform for push-off. When the second metatarsal (or, less commonly, the first) is longer (B), an unstable, single point of contact is created prior to push-off, encouraging the foot to progress more medially or laterally.

Imbalances can also be created through changes in the soft tissue, especially with a high arch pattern and short plantar fascia. This functional (rather than structural) imbalance can often cause the push-off to occur over the third, fourth, and fifth metatarsal heads rather than the first and second. This leads to a reduction in the amount of power produced in the myofascial trigger of the SBL, which may have to be compensated for by more work being produced elsewhere—often in the hip flexors.

Push-off on the medial aspect of the big toe can lead to the development of hallux valgus (bunion), and without sagittal plane progression over the first and second toes, torsion forces may be produced at the knee, causing a knee valgus pattern and thus creating issues for the ligaments (especially medial) and/or the menisci (lateral) (see fig. 3.20).

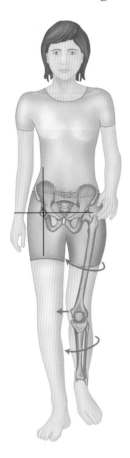

Figure 3.20. Pushing off via the medial aspect of the big toe creates torsional forces for the first metatarsophalangeal joint (usually leading to hallux valgus) and a valgus force at the knee. This can lead to increased strain on the medial ligaments, due to the opening of the joint on the medial side, along with the possible compression of the lateral meniscus, due to the closing of the joint on that side.

This dynamic can be exaggerated by wearing shoes with pointed or restricted toe boxes. Crushing the phalanges can mechanically misalign the foot, leading to further joint distress with the added forces of walking. A wide toe box, which allows the metatarsals to spread, is ideal, not just for the joint alignment, but also to stimulate the interossei, which have a reflex relationship with the quadriceps. As the metatarsals spread, mechanoreceptors in the tissue between them sense the movement and relay the impulse to the knee extensors to absorb the forces of gravity and ground reaction force (Michaud 2011).

Pushing off is most efficient if done on a platform of two metatarsal heads, and these will need to be in alignment in the sagittal and the frontal planes. Unfortunately, another common metatarsal misalignment is a "plantarflexed first ray" (the ray being the line of bones of the first metatarsal and medial cuneiform). This is apparent when the head of the first metatarsal remains below the line of the others when the foot is held in neutral. The effect on the frontal plane rocker depends on whether the first ray is mobile, semiflexible, or fixed. If the ray is fixed in plantarflexion, it will force the foot to supinate and push-off laterally. If it is mobile, the foot will be more likely to roll medially and into pronation (possibly encouraging a hallux valgus). A semiflexible first ray is less traumatic for the rest of the foot biomechanics but can lead to more impact to the sesamoid bones if the first ray is unable to rise enough on impact.

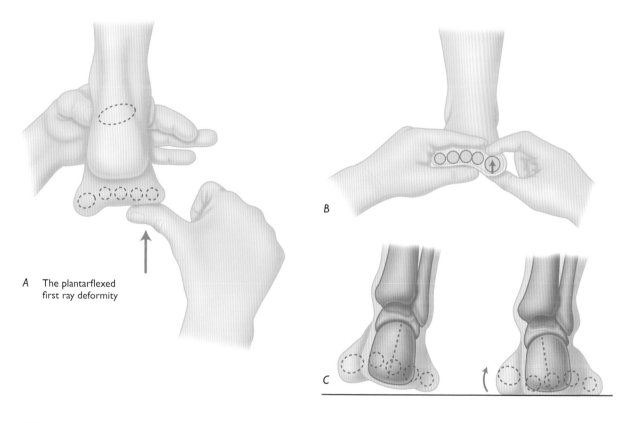

A   The plantarflexed
    first ray deformity

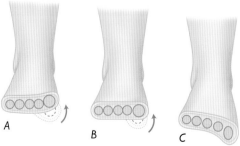

Figure 3.21.A, When the foot is aligned in neutral and the first ray remains below the level of the others, it should be checked for mobility (B). If it is hypermobile and rises above the level of the others, it can create instability of the first ray and lead to pronation. If it is fixed, the reverse will occur, and the foot will progress into supination as it is forced laterally. When the first metatarsal is only semimobile, coming into line with the others, impact forces will be transferred to the underlying sesamoids, creating inflammation that may lead to other compensations and limping. Resolution of these patterns may involve the peroneus longus muscle, as well as manipulation of the joints, if they are restricted. Adapted from Michaud, 2011.

Toe Rocker

The first and second metatarsophalangeal joints must be in balance with one another and must be able to reach 40 to 55 degrees of extension. Any reduction in this ability will again lead to compensations, usually within the transverse plane.

"Hallux rigidus" is a fusion at the first metatarsophalangeal joint with little possibility of correction and therefore requires adaptation of the environment—either footwear or use of orthotics.

"Hallux limitus" simply refers to any reduction in extension ability of the big toe below the 40- to 45-degree ideal necessary for push-off. The reasons for its development may be many, and full orthopedic investigation may be required to check for bony changes. Manipulative intervention can include treatment of any and all of the big toe flexors, especially the flexor hallucis brevis.

Knee Extension

As the leg swings through before heel strike, the knee will gradually come into extension. We will revisit this in chapters 5 and 6 ("Spiral Line" and "Deep Front Line"), where we will see that knee extension allows for communication between the biceps femoris and the fibularis muscles (SPL), and between the adductor magnus and the deep posterior compartment (DFL). Knee extension may also be a useful addition to help distribute some of the contraction force from the hamstrings. The hamstrings' interlocking with the tissue of the gastrocnemius at the moment of heel strike allows the calf tissue to help stabilize the limb and absorb some of the force. As a bonus, it might help initiate knee flexion, along with the force of gravity.

Immediately after heel strike, the knee will flex by approximately 20 to 25 degrees to absorb the associated forces, and then gradually straighten again prior to heel lift. As discussed above, the flexion will assist with the extension, through the recoil of elastic energy, and then, once the leg is straight, other body segments can communicate force across the knee and allow the knee extensors to be relatively passive.

It has been found that walking with a knee-bent gait leads to an increased usage of oxygen by up to 50 percent, showing the extent of the inefficiency of this gait, compared to allowing the knee to fully extend (Michaud 2011). This is further evidenced by the differences in strength between the other primates and humans. The average chimp is much stronger than the average human; this is caused by a combination of genetic variance and muscle architecture. While chimps also have pennate muscles—muscles with fibers aligned at an angle to the line of pull, which increases muscle efficiency—

their fibers tend to be longer, allowing them to produce more power over a greater range. Chimps also have higher levels of a gene called ACTN3, which creates more muscular muscles. In humans, ACTN3 is found in higher levels in sprinters and much lower in endurance runners. Therefore, it may be related to the fascial/muscle fiber balance within the soft tissues (Hawks 2009).

Possessing these differences allows the chimp and other apes to be comfortable walking with bent knees and hips.

Prior to heel lift, the knee flexes and the foot plantarflexes simultaneously, and it appears that we use the gastrocnemius to control both of these events: the power will be assisted by many other myofascial elements, but the coordination between these two events is strongly influenced by the "express" of the calf muscle. Factors that limit the extension of the knee could include lack of range in the gastrocnemius, chronic contracture of the hamstrings, and joint dysfunctions involving the menisci, cartilage, or ligaments. These can be tested by using a range of loaded and unloaded assessments to differentiate the tissues that may be involved.

Hip Extension/Flexion

Extension at the hip joint is restricted to approximately 10 degrees, due to the strong iliofemoral ligament, so to increase the length of the step, we use a blend of pelvic tilt and rotation in combination with hip extension (see fig. 3.22). By extending the hip, we will engage the iliofemoral ligament and the rectus femoris, and we will draw on the fascia of the upper SFL, meaning that the tissue of the rectus abdominis helps with hip flexion (see exercise 3.4).

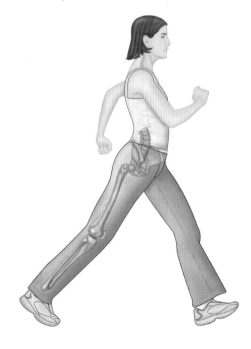

Figure 3.22. The apparent extension of the hip is partially created by the pelvis tilting and rotating. Limitations in hip extension will often force the pelvis to tilt or rotate farther, probably increasing the stresses on the lumbar and thoracic spine. Limitation in hip extension can also lead to a shorter stride, which may fail to rotate and torsion the pelvis, reducing the elastic loading of the other myofascial lines in the upper body and thereby increasing the work being done by the leg (including the psoas).

Lack of hip flexion will limit the amount of pre-tensioning placed on the SBL (as well as the Back Functional Line, the Spiral Line, and the posterior section of the Deep Front Line). Lack of hip flexion, however, will also reduce the lever created at heel strike, as the foot will be placed closer to the body's center of gravity and therefore will require less work to be done to resist gravity and produce hip extension. This will force the posterior chain muscles to work harder, and the gait will look labored, compared to the ease of someone fully engaging his or her fascial spring mechanisms.

The use of the springs of the SFL and SBL allow minimal contractions in hip and knee muscles and, if orchestrated correctly, the foot progresses with just 1.29 centimeters of ground clearance (Michaud 2011). The range of each of the lower limb flexions are kept small, and they are not consciously created but produced by the release of the "trigger" of the toe rocker. One quickly feels the difference between walking on a smooth surface and an uneven surface that requires greater ground clearance and, therefore, more muscle effort.

Lumbar Extension

As discussed above, lumbar extension is one of the unique human traits that allow a bipedal gait, because it allows us to stand upright and also allows the pelvis to tilt anteriorly as we step forward. If the lumbars are extended due to an anteriorly tilted pelvis or a posteriorly tilted rib cage, they may limit the amount the client is able to extend his or her hip and draw on the front of the pelvis (see fig. 3.23).

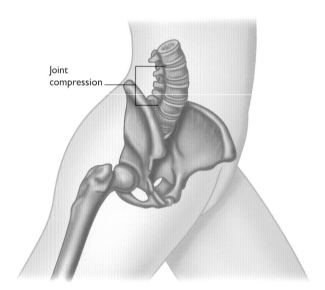

Figure 3.23. An anteriorly titled pelvis leads to further lumbar extension, which may reduce the amount of available hip extension, if the hip flexors are shorter than normal. The relative range of motion may also adjust to produce the appearance of greater range in extension and a limitation in flexion. The therapist's attention should first be on repositioning the pelvis rather than on hip flexor/extensor balance, provided that resting lengths are within normal limits.

Conversely, an anteriorly tilted pelvis may help with more apparent extension. If the hip flexors are of normal length and the orientation of the pelvis changes, then the range of movement, while not increasing in real terms, moves further into extension relative to the trunk and decreases the amount of apparent hip flexion. This can create a gait that looks longer in extension and shorter in flexion.

Thoracic Extension and Head Position

Exercise 3.1 also demonstrated the relationship of head and trunk position to the power of or connection to leg flexion. An anterior head position and/or limited extension in the thoracic spine should also be addressed to reduce strain in the deep hip flexors. If the SFL cannot fully and properly engage, hip flexion may be initiated from the Deep Front Line instead, leading to overuse.

The structural issues above may be produced by an overly short SFL, drawing the head down and compressing the front of the rib cage, in which case the superficial tissues may engage quite early in hip extension. If the client is unable to fully extend the hip, the Deep Front Line may not be correctly loaded and will be unable to assist with the flexion. This scenario could lead to overuse of the SFL or to a rotational strategy, in which the client turns the limb (internally or externally) to avoid the limitation of the SFL/SBL. This rotational compensation could be used ameliorate any of the sagittal plane events, especially at the foot and the hip. When medial or lateral deviations are noticed (especially when they are more apparent functionally compared to structurally), each of these sagittal plane "essential events" should be assessed for range and quality of motion.

SUMMARY

Each of these sagittal plane "essential events" is necessary for full involvement of the SFL and SBL, allowing them to utilize the full potential energy created by fascial lengthening.

In developing an upright, bipedal gait, our alignment with gravity became more centralized than that of quadrupeds and the primate knuckle walkers. While it has produced the need for greater stability, it has also given us the ability to use forward movement to load the fascial continuities with elastic energy. It is as if our skeleton stretches the fascial lines by walking into them, the pelvis pushing back or forward to create length and the muscles adjusting the tension to minimize the work involved in keeping us upright and moving forward.

Gravity loads the tissue in response to the resistance of ground reaction forces, and the propulsion forward or backward creates slings to catapult us forward. These elastic, myofascial catapults are controlled by certain triggers, the greatest one being push-off at the toes, which releases the energy simultaneously from both the middle portion of the SFL and the lower portion of the SBL.

As we will see, the pelvic and hip joints also create elastic loading for other continuities in the frontal (Lateral Line) and transverse planes (Spiral and Functional Lines), with the Deep Front Line being assisted by all three planes. Once we have these in balance, we can really gain the "spring in our step."

4 Lateral Line

Happy is the man who has acquired the love of walking for its own sake!
—W.J. Holland

INTRODUCTION

Brain size is often used as a species indicator by scientists studying the ancestral hominid lineage. Along with other morphological indicators, brain size has been used to differentiate the *Homo* genus from the earlier *Australopithecus*—and from *Ardipithecus* before them (see fig. 4.1). Few people realize, however, that our extinct cousins, the Neanderthals—with whom we shared the world for around three hundred thousand years—not only had larger, more muscular bodies than *Homo sapiens* but also had larger brains. Why, then, were we able to outlast our brainier and brawnier cohabitants?

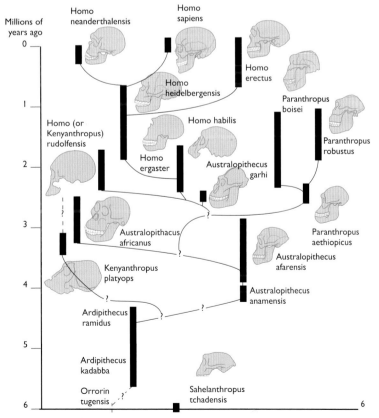

Figure 4.1. A hypothetical hominin family tree.

In *Anatomy Trains,* Myers describes how the multipurpose sensory organs of the ear lie along our lateral aspects (2009). This could be where we had our competitive advantage. As Myers and McCredie point out, the sides of our bodies have their evolutionary origin in the lateral line organs of fish, which are used to perceive vibrations from the surrounding environment (Myers 2009; McCredie 2007). These piscine sensory organs evolved into the human ear, with its ability not only to hear but also to sense orientation and movement: the semicircular canals of the inner ear can perceive the three dimensions: pitch, roll, and yaw.

Recent investigations on Neanderthal skulls have shown that their semicircular canals were smaller and less developed than those of *Homo sapiens.* Balance, coordination, running, and throwing would presumably have been more difficult for them (but by no means impossible). Analysis of Neanderthal skeletons shows the kind of wear and tear, injuries and arthroses experienced by today's rodeo riders, presumably caused by the need to get close enough to their prey to jab them with spears (McCredie 2007; Wynn and Coolidge 2012).

Compare that to the picture of *Homo sapiens* painted by Bramble and Lieberman and by McDougall, of a graceful and elegant distance runner bounding from boulder to boulder and hurdling tree roots (Bramble and Lieberman 2004; McDougall 2010). A great level of balance and coordination is required for persistence hunting (chasing the prey to exhaustion and death, which Lieberman and McDougall propose many modern hunter-gatherers excel at) and for the accurate throwing of spears and shooting of arrows. It has been proposed that humans' superior inner-ear apparatus gave us all of these abilities, as well as enhanced navigational skills. The ability to find our way back to camp after chasing an antelope for many miles would be an essential element in the toolbox of a persistence hunter, and this is certainly enabled by a larger inner ear. The evidence of Neanderthal lifestyle seems to show they rarely traveled far from their main encampment (Wynn and Coolidge 2012).

Furthermore, having a better developed proprioceptive sense (the perception of where one's body is in space) allows our brains to carry on with other jobs, as we no longer have to pay as much conscious attention to the surrounding environment and our relationship to it. This is exemplified by the case of Ian Waterman, a man whose brain lost the ability to receive many of nerve signals from his body—while not paralyzed, he could not feel his body's existence and could not instinctively move it. Mr. Waterman was able to teach himself how to walk again, but walking required his full concentration and reliance on visual input; when distracted, he would fall; trying to move in the dark would be impossible (Muller and Schleip 2011).

Perhaps *Homo sapiens* was able to find an effective (I hesitate to say "ideal") balance between brain and brawn by developing our proprioceptive and coordinating abilities. Evolution and function are difficult to tie down to just a handful of factors, as many serendipitous and contingent evolutionary events were required for our ability to walk, talk, and throw all at the same time. However, the increase in the functional ability of our inner-ear system must have contributed significantly. It allowed us to take advantage of our elastic tissue, since moving elastically requires more deviation from the midline and allows us to use the momentum of our bodies in different ways, as in gymnastics or parkour. Furthermore, the less we have to think about moving, the better we will be at the many other requirements of life, adding to our efficiency. Having less brain processing tied up with spatial awareness is likely to have given us more adaptability.

It is estimated that the average calorie intake of Neanderthals, with their heavy, muscular build and large bones, would have been between 3,500 and 5,500 calories per day, mostly gained from a variety of meat sources (Wynn and Coolidge 2012). It is easy to extrapolate that our lighter and more elastic frames required a lower daily calorie intake (2,000 to 3,000), while our greater spatial awareness gifted us with both a wider range of movement and the ability to maintain larger territorial maps in our minds. In essence, the combination of our inner-ear advances and our lighter frames gave us strong evolutionary advantages.

THE STABILIZING LINE

Some folks look at me and see a certain swagger, which in Texas is called *walking*.
—George W. Bush

The adaptation of the inner ear is not the only aspect of the lateral line to contribute to our bipedal success. As we saw earlier, standing on one leg requires the ilia to face laterally to provide frontal-plane stability. Our femur's angle inward from the hip to the knee allows us to align our feet more directly under our center of gravity (see fig. 4.3, overleaf). We work against gravity in other ways as well. When we walk, the position of our feet moves inward closer to our center of gravity than they are when we are in our "anatomical neutral" (i.e., standing upright), and in addition, we shift our body weight laterally as we step. This pushes the greater trochanter out against the band of tissue of the Lateral Line, whose most obvious role in walking is in supporting the pelvis in the frontal plane. The deltoid of the hip abductors (tensor fascia lata, gluteus medius, and gluteus maximus) are called into play, preventing the pelvis from dropping too far into adduction at heel strike and into the swing phase, when the body weight is carried on one limb (see fig. 4.3, overleaf). The knack is making sure that the "swagger" is controlled enough and doesn't become too "Texan."

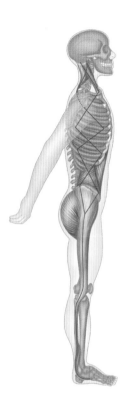

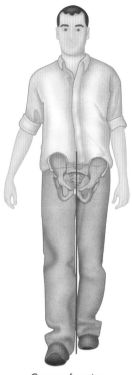

Center of gravity

Figure 4.2. The Lateral Line.

Figure 4.3. One of the main strategies the body uses to minimize the effort of bipedal gait is a side swing toward the weight-bearing foot. The combination of this movement and the acceptance of the body weight onto the foot causes the pelvis to drop slightly on the non-weight-bearing side. This passively adducts the hip joint on the weight-bearing side, loading the Lateral Line tissues.

The shifting of the greater trochanter into the Lateral Line stretches it from the inside (see fig. 4.3). Tautening this supportive band of fascia, controlled by the gluteus maximus and gluteus medius (both of which are tensioned to decelerate the flexion and adduction of the hip) and the tensor fascia lata (tensioned to control adduction), adds stiffness to this line. Each event assists the other—the contraction of the muscles tightens the fascia, the tightening of the fascia created by the lateral sway assists the integrity of the muscular contraction.

This combined strategy of shifting the weight to the stance side and allowing the hip joint to adduct reduces the forces that have to be carried by the abductors. This section of the lateral line works as a "hydraulic amplifier": the fascia lata, stretched tight over the muscles—like shrink wrapping—helps to disperse the force through a greater proportion of tissue (for more, see "Hydraulic Amplifiers" in chapter 5). The sway to the side will push the thigh and pelvis out against the tissue of the lower portion of the Lateral Line, passively increasing the fascial tension throughout the more superficial fascial layers of the thigh and pelvic area on the weight-bearing side. The deeper tissue of the quadriceps and hamstrings expand outward, pressing on the "shrink wrapping" of the fascia lata, and so the area works together, as a system, rather than as individual parts. This is in contrast to the traditional presentation of the thigh (as shown in fig 4.3), which focuses the deceleration forces from the hip joint onto the attachment of the iliotibial band.

As with most of the other lines, tension is not consistent along the Lateral Lines through the phases of gait. In figure 4.3, the iliac crest is moving away from the femur on the right (the heel-strike side), while on the other side, the ilium and the rib cage are separating.

This book analyzes each line—and therefore each plane of movement—in turn, but it is important to keep in mind that events occur simultaneously in all three planes. For example, the left ilium is supported in all three planes of motion by a variety of lines (see fig. 4.4). The natural movement of the pelvis, created by the action of the lower limbs, creates these lines of tension, which are controlled by myofascial chains. Though this book concentrates on one plane at a time, hopefully, as we add the other lines to the picture, a full three-dimensional image will come into focus.

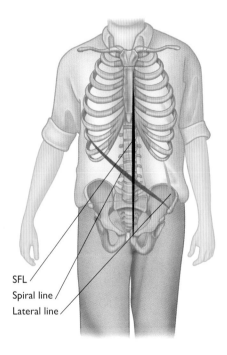

SFL
Spiral line
Lateral line

Figure 4.4. Following heel strike, the ilium of the opposite limb (shown here as the figure's left side) will be anteriorly and inferiorly tilted and rotated. These movements are controlled/decelerated by the SFL, LTL, and SPL, respectively.

Foot Eversion/Inversion and the Rockers

The lower portion of the Lateral Line works hardest from heel strike to weight acceptance, with the large deltoid of hip abductors contracting strongly to prevent too much adduction and gluteus maximus assisting the control of femoral rotation and further hip flexion (more on this in chapter 5). If we follow this lateral force down the leg along the Lateral Line, some of it should cross over the head of the fibula and affect the fibularis longus and brevis.

It is possible that some of the force of the strong contraction of the iliotibial tract helps the foot adapt to the ground on heel strike. The fibularis longus could assist the fall of the medial arch, and the fibularis brevis may pull the base of the fifth metatarsal—and thereby the forefoot—into a lateral rotation (see fig. 4.5).

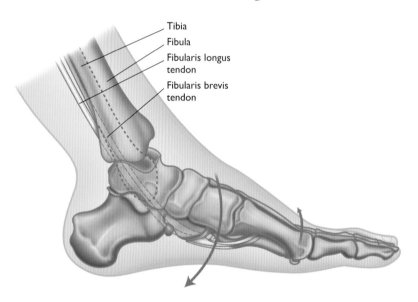

Tibia
Fibula
Fibularis longus tendon
Fibularis brevis tendon

Figure 4.5. Any force that comes along the fascia of the Lateral Line and into the fascial tissue of fibularis longus and brevis may help the foot adapt to the ground. The fibularis longus may help the medial tilt of the medial cuneiform and first metatarsal, while fibularis brevis encourages the forefoot to laterally rotate, via its insertion into the base of the fifth metatarsal.

Whether this transfer of force from the iliotibial band actually occurs has yet to be established (the transfer of force/strain from biceps femoris to the lateral compartment is suggested by a study performed by Franklyn-Miller in 2009, but this does not necessarily mean the same for the iliotibial band). Nevertheless, the lengthening of the fibularis tissue must take place if the foot is then to correct itself from its pronation and adaptation to the ground. As the rest of the limb progresses through the ankle and foot rockers (see figs. 4.5 and 4.6), the dorsiflexion that occurs will require the tissue of both fibularis muscles to be free from tethering (i.e., they must be free to glide through their associated retinaculum), and they must be long enough for the medial arch to lift again, which will allow the forefoot to come back in line with the calcaneus (see fig. 4.6).

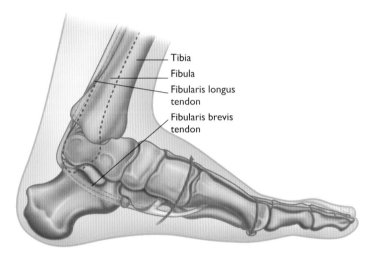

Figure 4.6. Once the ankle comes into dorsflexion, the foot must be assisted back to its neutral position from its pronated position (this will partially be done via the SPL and DFL). This supination of the foot requires lengthening of the fibularis tissue to bring the foot back from the lateral rotation and medial tilt. The fascia of the fibularii is able to relax as the strain transferred down from the hip abductors is gradually unloaded by the body first coming into line above the foot and then heel striking on the opposite side.

A restriction of dorsiflexion, whether due to a block of the anterior joint or a constriction of the Achilles tendon or posterior compartment, can lead to an exaggerated gait with the toes pointed out. Differential diagnosis of some form is required to find the culprit; often it is due to the commonly overlooked fibularis compartment. Even if the fibularis muscles were not the original cause, if the foot is not combining dorsiflexion with inversion, these muscles may not get challenged to their end of range and thus may develop a functional shortness, thereby becoming part of the problem. Exercises and stretches that combine these motions should be included in most foot and ankle routines (if safe to do so).

Salsa! The Lateral Line and Side Flexion of the Spine

The tilt of the pelvis helps to stimulate the abdominals, and it also requires an adaptation in the spine. If we look at the lateral flexion ability of each segment of the spine on the spinal movement chart (fig. 4.7), we see that the lower lumbars have a gradual increase in lateral flexibility up to L3/L4.

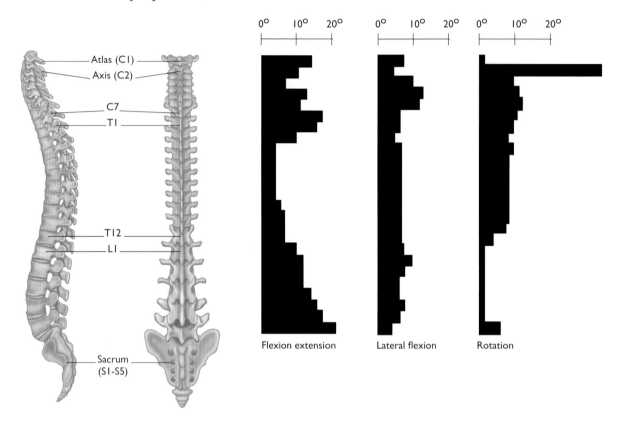

Figure 4.7. For head stability, the spine must adapt to and diminish movement on the three planes of movement occurring in the pelvis. Much of the lateral tilt (a frontal plane movement) is dealt with by the lower lumbars, L3 and below. The chart shows a gradual increase in side flexion ability from L5/S1 up to L3/L4, a slight decrease in the mid-lumbars, and another increase around the thoracolumbar junction. Side flexion ability stays relatively consistent throughout the thoracics until the cervico-thoracic junction. (Adapted from Middleditch and Oliver 2005.)

The side flexion of the lowest lumbars lets the spine mimic a tree growing on a hillside. The lower part of the trunk will adapt its growth to send the rest of the tree skyward (see fig. 4.8A). The lower lumbar area absorbs the frontal plane movement of the pelvis, with the iliolumbar fibers of the quadratus lumborum correcting the tilt of the pelvis and the iliolumbar ligament preventing further hip adduction (see fig. 4.8B). If this system loses some of its adaptability, the tilt may be forced up to the thoracolumbar junction, which also allows side flexion (see fig. 4.4), before reaching the vertebrae of the less flexible thoracic cage.

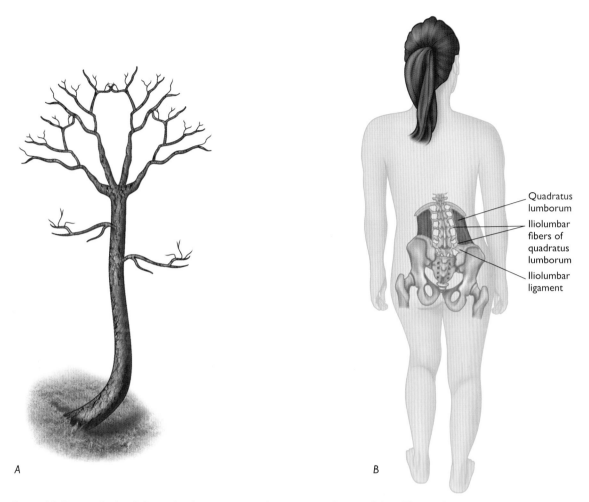

A   *B*

Figure 4.8. Keeping the head skyward and minimizing its tilt requires a reduction of the adduction that occurs at the hip in natural gait. Like the bend of the tree trunk (A), most of the deviation of the pelvis in frontal plane movement can be absorbed early in the spine if the movement is allowed by the iliolumbar ligaments and the iliolumbar fibers of the quadratus lumborum (B). If it is not, the side flexion will travel higher (as we saw with the rotation) and can create—or demand—a hypermobility around the thoracolumbar junction.

Clinical Note

A simple test for the ability of the pelvis to drop away from the lower rather than the upper lumbars is to have your client stand in front of you and bend one knee. Ask him or her to keep both feet on the floor, and the foot on the target side will naturally roll forward on the ankle or forefoot rocker (see fig. 4.9A). This will cause the pelvis to drop on one side, and the bend should occur predominately in the section of the spine below L3 (see fig. 4.9B).

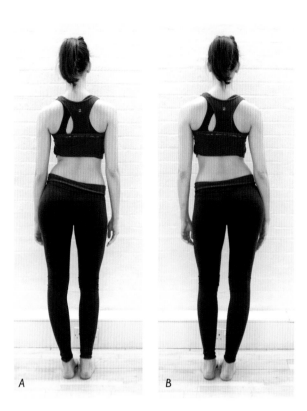

Figure 4.9. Ask your client to stand with feet hip-width apart and roughly parallel, and then simply bend one knee, keeping the foot on the floor (A). This will cause the pelvis to drop on the side of the forward knee, and the freedom of the lumbars on the opposite side can be assessed. A responsive spine will show a clear lateral bend before L3 (B), one that is unable to absorb the movement in the lower lumbars will force the bend to occur higher in the spine.

The Xs of the Waist

Once above the waist, the Lateral Line travels upward in a series of crossed tissues (see fig. 4.2). This may seem contrary to Myers's rule that the Anatomy Trains travel in straight lines, but we will see that this provides a number of advantages and does not actually break the rule, as it is the combined vector of force between the muscular elements that maintains a vertical direction of contraction or support.

When the feet are at heel strike and push-off, the pelvis will be rotated toward the side of the extended leg, as described in chapter 3. This creates a relative rotation between the pelvis and the thorax, and therefore, the direction of force required for stability between the pelvis and the rib cage will not be truly vertical but will be at an oblique angle (see fig. 4.10). The Spiral Line (from the anterior superior iliac spine to the opposite shoulder girdle) and Functional Line (from the pubic ramus to the opposite humerus) play roles in supporting the ilium on the push-off/swing side. The Lateral Lines assist the work of these other lines in producing and controlling rotation, but they also offer frontal plane stability by providing varying amounts of oblique lines of force. The oblique angles of the Lateral Lines are therefore essential: if there were only vertically aligned lines, the relative rotation between the pelvis and the thorax would lead to a great deal of instability. The X arrangement of the Lateral Lines thereby maintains the body's ability to rotate but still retain left/right integrity.

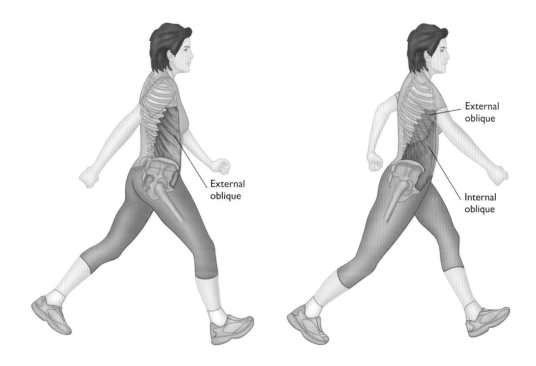

Figure 4.10. At full stride, there is a relative rotation between the pelvis and the thorax, which is controlled (and also limited!) by the alternate obliques on either side. This arrangement allows the body to be stable in the frontal plane by contracting different proportions of the internal and external obliques on both sides.

The oblique muscles also affect and are affected by the length of stride, either decelerating or limiting the amount of rotation between the thorax and pelvis as we reach full stride length. Therefore, if a client shows the thorax and pelvis rotating at the same or a similar rate—or if one shows a limited stride length (which would serve to minimize rotation)—the range of motion of the obliques should be examined.

The "Fish Body" and the Intercostals

The upper portion of the Lateral Line follows along the rib cage with the external and internal intercostals, which, like the obliques, are oriented at angles. This brings them into play with the rotation that travels through the thorax in movement, performing a role between each rib similar to that performed by the obliques between the costal arch and the iliac crest: controlling the relative rotation between each section.

Because of this arrangement, the intercostals are sometimes thought to be as involved with walking as they are with breathing. Like the obliques, they help the Functional and Spiral Lines deal with transverse plane movement, acting like a watch spring: they wind up in one direction to uncoil in the other. We will see this mechanism again in chapter 5, on the Spiral Line, though the Spiral Line operates on a more superficial layer. This demonstrates the difference between the "fish body" and the evolutionarily "new" body, which includes the shoulder girdle.

As the Lateral Line moves up the rib cage, it follows a line deep to the tissue of the arms and shoulder girdles (see fig. 4.11)—the "fish body." Being on a deeper layer of tissue keeps the Lateral Line—which works toward the stability of the trunk—separate from the multidirectional lines of mobility for the arms and shoulders (part of the "new" body), which begin on the trunk with the pectorals, latissimus dorsi, and rhomboids, all of which are superficial to and glide over the rib cage. This leads us to an important concept of the separation of different vectors of force, which we will see further with the Spiral Line and the ways in which we use the shoulder girdles to stabilize the head when the trunk is moving, such as in walking. The Lateral Line is very much involved with providing lower cervical stabilization in the frontal plane.

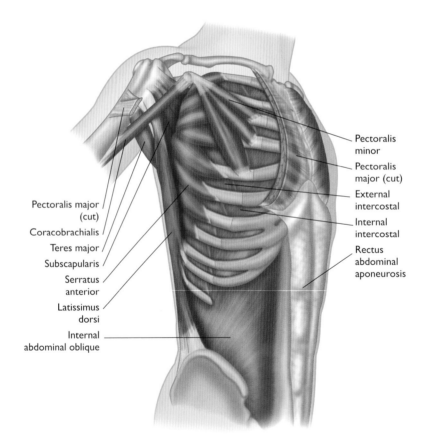

Figure 4.11. From this view, we can see the intercostals are on a separate level from the myofascia traveling to the shoulder. This allows a differentiation of force transfer: the deeper Lateral Line will carry a smaller range of motion, while the more superficial tissues go through a wider movement.

CERVICAL STABILITY

The Lateral Lines continue from the intercostals to the cervical spine via the scalenes. Myers uses the sternal portion of the sternocleidomastoid and the splenius capitis to bring this line to the cranium, claiming that these two muscles create stability for the head. In standing, this may well be true, but I believe the arms and shoulders come into play much more during movement. The weight of the upper girdles is used to counterbalance the head, and they combine a variety of strategies to help keep the head upright and supported (see chapter 5).

I prefer to track the upper portion of the Lateral Line to C2/C3 via the scalenes (see fig. 4.2). When we look at the chart of spinal movements (see fig. 4.7), we can divide the cervicals into two sections: the upper portion, C2 to the occiput, is the more mobile; the lower portion, C7 to C3, is less so. The lower section still has a comparatively large range of motion, but nothing compared to the rotation of C1/C2 and the flexion/extension of the atlanto-occipital joint. In terms of the functional, moving body, the Lateral Lines give support to the lower, more stabile portion of the neck, up to C3. The upper cervicals to the occiput are free from the strong tethers of the scalene muscles to perform fine adjustments to keep the eyes and ears oriented to the horizon. This arrangement allows the head to be independent from overly stabilizing forces (see fig. 4.12).

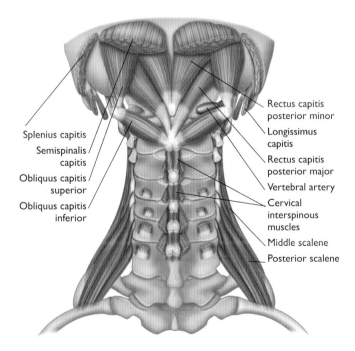

Splenius capitis
Semispinalis capitis
Obliquus capitis superior
Obliquus capitis inferior

Rectus capitis posterior minor
Longissimus capitis
Rectus capitis posterior major
Vertebral artery
Cervical interspinous muscles
Middle scalene
Posterior scalene

Figure 4.12. Here we can see how the lower, stabile portion of the neck is strongly tethered to the rib cage by the scalenes, which form an anchoring skirt of support for the cervicals up to C2/C3 in each of the three planes of motion. C2 to the occiput has a much larger variety of smaller, "local" (one- and two-joint) muscles, which give fine control to the occiput, atlas, and axis complex.

By extending the Lateral Line to the scalenes rather than to the splenius capitis and sternocleidomastoid, we stay true to the "fish body," as we remain on the same myofascial layer. As we will see in the next chapter, the more superficial myofascial layers developed at a later stage, when the head separated from the rib cage by developing the cervical spine, a stage of evolution that coincided with the increase in the size and development of the shoulder girdles and their associated musculature.

SUMMARY

1. The Lateral Line gives frontal plane stability to allow for the single-leg stance, an ability brought about by the evolutionary change in the orientation of the ilium.

2. To ease the load on the abductors, we naturally swing our pelvis to the side of the stance leg, bringing our center of gravity over the base of support, the stance foot, and minimizing the work of maintaining balance.

3. The movement of the pelvis and the adduction of the hip helps to load the fascial tissue of the Lateral Lines in the frontal plane, thereby increasing its efficiency and assisting with the recoil back to neutral.

4. The loading of the abductors may increase the pronation of the foot by pulling on the fibularis muscles, which will then have to release and lengthen to allow the foot to supinate and dorsiflex prior to push-off.

5. The rotation of the pelvis, produced by the SFL and SBL, will carry the rotation to the rib cage and into the intercostals to create a watch-spring mechanism for some of the rotational movement through the body.

6. The scalenes provide the internal stability lines for the lower and mid-neck, leaving the sub-occipitals free to provide for last-minute and fine adjustment of head stabilization, and thereby differentiating the "fish body" from the cranium.

ESSENTIAL EVENTS

Frontal Plane Adjustment

The most obvious first feature of the Lateral Line is its ability to deal with the frontal plane loads. The client should be able to displace his or her body weight over the supporting foot to realign the center of gravity, and the hip should be able to adduct by approximately 4 degrees.

The maintenance of the center of gravity over the feet is facilitated by a number of mechanisms. The first is the evolutionary adaptation that has angled the femur inward, requiring the medial condyle to be larger than the lateral in order for them both to rest on the plateau of the more vertically aligned tibia (see fig. 4.13).

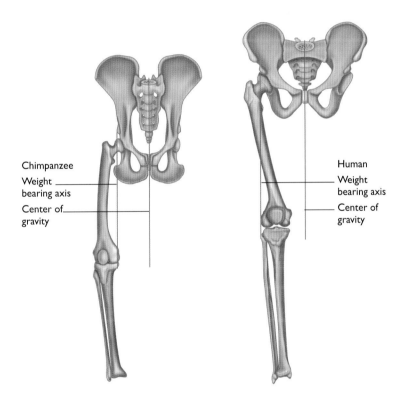

Chimpanzee
Weight
bearing axis
Center of
gravity

Human
Weight
bearing axis
Center of
gravity

Figure 4.13. Human legs are less vertically oriented below the hip joint than those of other primates. This allows our support to be closer to the center of gravity and leads to the adaptation of the enlarged medial condyle—a feature that is developed by walking rather than being inherited.

The abductors must therefore be both strong enough to deal with the weight and long enough to allow the transfer and adduction to occur. Without this happening, the abdominals on the opposite side will not lengthen in the frontal plane, which would diminish their efficiency in dealing with rotation.

The lumbar spine must be able to cope with the side flexion in its lower portion (S1–L3), otherwise the lateral deviation will be sent to the thoracolumbar junction, causing overextension and overuse (as addressed in the "Clinical Notes" above). Decreased mobility in the lumbars or stiffness in the hip abductors can lead to upper-body sway, as the client will find it difficult to differentiate between the pelvis and the rib cage, causing the two to move together and bringing the whole body over the supporting foot.

There is also a contralateral relationship between the hip abductors on one side and the adductors of the opposite. For the pelvis to tilt, both have to be able to lengthen, so for the Lateral Line to truly load in the frontal plane, the clinician needs to check at least three areas—the hip abductors, adductors, and the lower lumbar spine (see fig. 4.14).

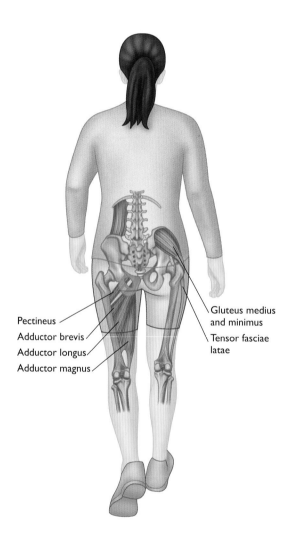

Pectineus
Adductor brevis
Adductor longus
Adductor magnus

Gluteus medius
and minimus
Tensor fasciae
latae

Figure 4.14. The side sway and hip adduction following heel strike requires at least three areas of adaptation. The hip abductors on the forward limb must lengthen to allow the pelvis to drop, an action also facilitated by the hip adductors on the other leg. If the pelvis tilts, the lower lumbars should be able to absorb some of that movement in its lower section to remove some stress from the thoracolumbar junction. The lumbar movement will be controlled by the iliolumbar fibers of the quadratus lumborum, but it could also be influenced by overly taught lateral abdominals. This triad of soft tissue is arranged in a triangular pattern.

Leg Length Differences

Leg length differences can also affect the movements of the pelvis. The client can be assessed by placing the medial malleoli together and having his or her knees bent. In this position, any structural length differences in the tibia or femur will be apparent (see fig. 4.15).

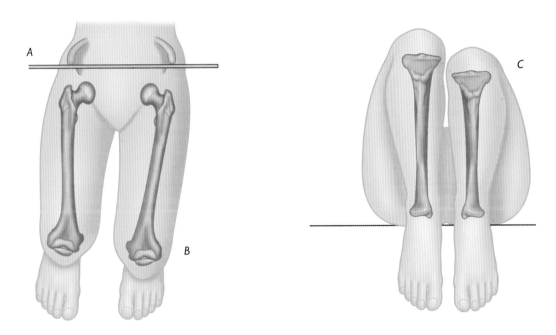

Figure 4.15. In this standard orthopedic test, ensure both ASIS are level and place the medial malleoli together to create a neutral (A). This will allow the therapist to assess the length of the femurs and the heights of the tibia. A longer femur will reveal itself by pushing the knee farther from the body (B), and a longer tibia will produce a higher tibial tuberosity or knee-joint line (C). It is important for the feet to be placed parallel to the pelvis and in the midline in order to read the legs in an anatomical neutral.

Any discrepancy in leg length can be compensated for by changes in the arches—the long leg may pronate or the shorter one supinate, or sometimes combination of the two—and these alterations can effectively balance the limbs. This can have implications for therapeutic input, as the compensations may be beneficial for the client. Thus any work with them should also ensure that the rest of the system is able to cope with the new positions.

Foot Balance

Changes in the feet can also lead to "apparent" differences in leg length. The leg may appear longer if the foot is more supinated, or it can appear shorter if the foot is pronated. These cases of functional leg-length difference may be easier to correct than dealing with real length differences, which will require a more detailed understanding of the many compensations that may have occurred in the client's body. Each case will require individual recommendations.

The fibularis muscles are essential to the correct functioning of the medial longitudinal arch. The fibularis longus is required to draw the first metatarsal into the medial cuneiform, balancing the pull of the tibialis anterior (we will see this relationship again in the sling of the Spiral Line). The fibularis brevis performs a similar role for the fifth metatarsal. If the brevis is unable to lengthen fully as the ankle dorsiflexes, it will keep the foot in a laterally rotated position, which often prevents the midtarsal joints from reengaging prior to push-off (see fig. 4.6).

Structural Shifts

A longer leg can create an angled sacral base, which the spine must adapt to by bending to one side. If the body is held long enough in a shifted position, it may adapt to that pattern by creating restricted or adhered tissue. A slight deviation in the lower spine can develop when a parent frequently carries his or her child on a raised hip, or if a person who drives for long periods sits with one hip raised on an angled car seat or with a wallet in the back pocket. This displacing of the body weight to one side may lead to further frontal-plane discrepancies in movement, and/or create limitations in gait due to restricted tissue.

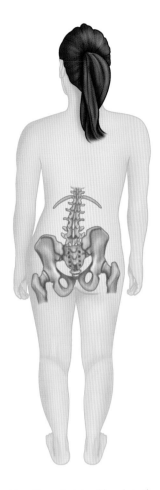

Figure 4.16. Having the sacral base angled to one side will create lateral bends in the spine. These can lead to tissue restrictions, especially around the iliolumbar ligament and the lower fibers of quadratus lumborum, and it may restrict the facet joint movement in the other planes.

Bends in the spine may also lead to restricted movement in the spinal facets, especially in the transverse plane. The closing of the articulations on one side of the vertebral column in the frontal plane will affect its ability to rotate, which can lead to many potential compensations—shorter strides, overextension in other spinal segments, or a lumbering side-to-side gait, as described above. Dealing with the structural issues first, by easing the side bends, prior to dealing with the functional issues can therefore be an appropriate strategy.[1]

1 For full descriptions on how to do this, see Earls and Myers, *Fascial Release for Structural Balance*, 2010.

Thoracic Rotation

The SBL and SFL create the relative rotation between the pelvis and the rib cage that allows the intercostals to contribute their energy to gait. For this to occur, there must be enough rotation between the two body segments to stretch and engage the thoracic musculature. This will require not only the spinal involvement described above but also the opposite-side internal and external obliques to be long enough and strong enough to carry the forces.

The ipsilateral oblique lines can be easily tested by having the client rotate his or her rib cage or lunge forward to assess the amount of available movement. Palpating the area as the client performs the test can give the necessary feedback, as the therapist will be able to feel if the obliques limit the movement or if they remain loose and uninvolved (see fig. 4.17).

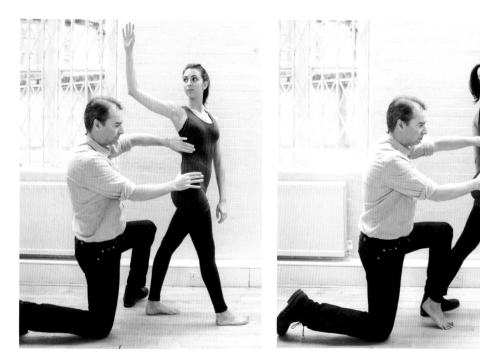

Figure 4.17. By palpating the muscles of the waist on both sides, the therapist can assess the range of motion and the amount of strength available from the obliques. Thoracic rotation and anterior lunging can be used while the therapist feels for any variation in quality between the external obliques on one side and the internal obliques on the other.

5 Spiral Line

It is a great art to saunter.
—Henry David Thoreau

INTRODUCTION

The Spiral Line is perhaps the line most involved throughout gait. It creates and decelerates the rotational forces of walking, absorbs some of the downward force of the body, and helps with flexion and extension. It can be one of the most confusing lines to follow, as it combines elements of sagittal and frontal plane movement with its obvious role in the transverse plane—thus involving itself in all three dimensions. Over the course of its length, the Spiral Line also progresses in depth, from the surface of the body to the interior, starting with the more superficial splenii muscles and ending at the head again with the deeper erectors. Passing through the shoulder girdle, it joins the axial to the appendicular skeletons, and it allows contralateral movement to occur between the upper and lower limbs, creating a meeting of rotational force somewhere between the two.

The Spiral Line is rarely tensioned along its full length at any one time. First we have to further define the different types of tensioning that can occur at various phases. Muscles can be contracting concentrically and eccentrically, and—somewhat confusingly—they can be lengthening at one end or in one plane and shortening at the other (Gray and Tiberio refer to this as "econcentric"). In this "econcentric" contraction, the muscle fiber is often acting predominately isometrically, and the movement of one bone (i.e., at one end of the muscle) is drawing the end of the muscle along with it. We see this in the tissue during dorsiflexion of the ankle and also in how the tensor fascia lata muscle will "lengthen" in hip extension but will simultaneously "shorten" with the internal rotation of the femur. Rethinking the eccentric/concentric or isometric model in this way allows us to see how bones can be affected not just by the movement of immediate neighbors but—using the Anatomy Trains lines—can also exploit the kinetic energy from more distant body parts.

Looking at the muscles in this way, we can see that they are not only actively working (i.e., contracting), but they are also adjusting the stiffness held within the system. Through experience, our bodies come to sense the ideal tension to hold that will allow the correct sequence of movement to occur and that will utilize the momentum from distant body parts to create desired effects. The muscles are therefore the tensioners within a "stiffness adjusting system," fine-tuning the correct amount of tension, either "gathering in" (concentric contraction) or "letting out" (eccentric contraction) in relation to the events all around, and allowing as much loading into the elastic fascial tissue as possible.

In this chapter, we will begin to see the hugely important contribution of the mechanoreceptors imbedded within the soft tissue: how they sense tension, movement, and shearing and relay this information to the surrounding tissue, striving for optimal efficiency.

The "Magpie"

The Spiral Line borrows muscles from many of the other lines, and—due to changes in direction and in ground reaction forces—it will take a few "switches," or junctions, that alter its path during a complete stride. These switches are created by the changes in mechanics, as the limbs and trunk shift direction from one phase to another. They will create a slightly different model when compared to the transfer of postural forces of someone standing still, and so we have to make a few alterations to Myers's classic Spiral Line to show its full involvement with function.

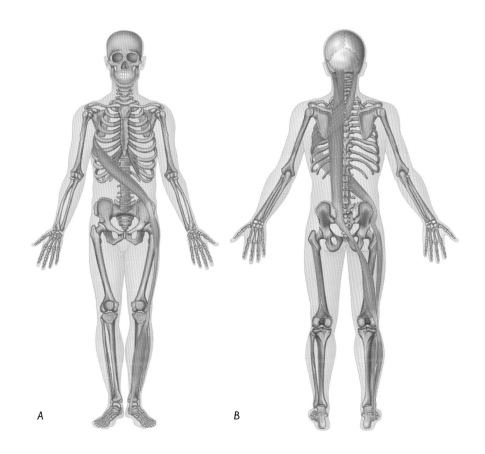

Figure 5.1.The Right Spiral Line, anterior (A) and posterior (B) views.

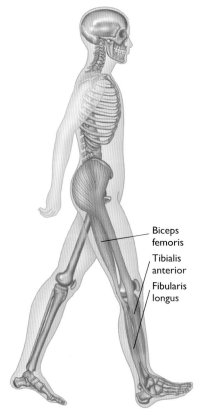

Biceps
femoris

Tibialis
anterior

Fibularis
longus

*Figure 5.2.We have to be a bit flexible with Myers's original description of the Spiral
Line.The transfer of structural forces are quite different once we come from the
anatomical position into movement, so we use a "switch" at the greater trochanter to
alter the line at heel strike.This recruits the gluteus maximus into the Spiral Line at heel
strike (in hip flexion) and the tensor fascia lata (when the hip progresses into extension,
not shown).This arrangement has cooperative influences through the rest of the body
for heel strike (at hip flexion) and push-off (at hip extension, see fig. 5.8).*

In chapter 2 we outlined the sequence of events following heel strike, a complex cascade of events taking place in all three planes of motion. So far we have dealt with the sagittal (SFL and SBL) and the frontal (LTL) planes, and now is the turn (if you excuse the pun) of the transverse. The rotation will turn on the body's obliquely oriented fibers, many of which we have already visited as part of the other lines. The Spiral Line's overlap with the other lines should not surprise us: transverse plane movement is a relatively new adaptation, one allowed in our primate heritage by the development of a long waist approximately 1.5 million years ago, first seen in fossils of *Homo ergaster.*

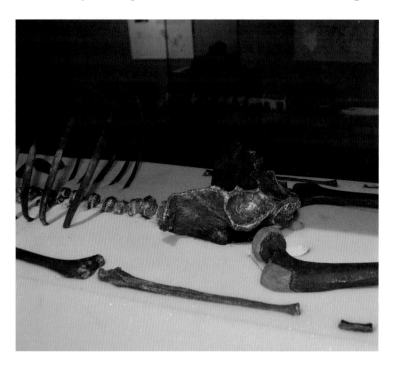

Figure 5.3. The long waist—seen here in the remains of "Turkana Boy," found in Kenya and dated to 1.5 MYA—shows the potential for counterrotation between the pelvis and the rib cage. Counterrotation is rarely seen in nonhuman primates, due to the shorter distance between these two body segments.

The many evolutionary changes in our skeletal structure and alignment were not always matched by changes in our musculature. The same muscles were present, they simply had their action and functions changed as they were forced to adapt to the new pathways forged within whichever skeletal "river beds" they ran through. Therefore, the development of the arch of the foot, the closer alignment of the big toe, the angulation of the femurs, and the relative independence between the thoracic cage and the pelvis introduced rotation and allowed the musculature to act in all three planes, rather than just two.

LOWER LIMB MECHANICS

Walking, as discussed earlier, is often described as "controlled falling," and, with one leg out in front of the body in mid-stride, it is easy to see why. The sequence of events following the pronation of the foot will have to be decelerated and controlled. Once the talus medially rotates and tilts on top of the calcaneus, it will bring the tibia and therefore the femur along with it, creating strong rotational forces at the joints (see chapter 2). If we follow the line of force along the lower limb, we come not to the tensor fascia lata (as in the classic Spiral Line) but to the gluteus maximus (see fig. 5.4).

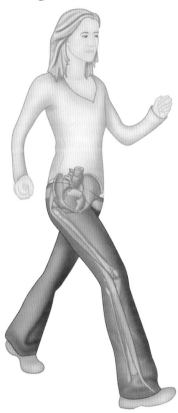

Figure 5.4. If we follow the internal rotation forces through the lower limb at heel strike, we come to the hip extensor side of the "hip deltoid" and into the gluteus maximus. We use the greater trochanter as a "switch" to include this hip extensor, which will work to prevent additional flexion at the joint. This gives us continuity in the lower limb from the gluteus maximus to the posterior portion of the iliotibial band, tibialis anterior, fibularis longus, and into the biceps femoris.

A lot of force is required to prevent the body from falling at heel strike, as the center of gravity is relatively far behind the point of support on the ground. Many muscles and Anatomy Trains lines will be involved in counteracting the downward force, but in particular, the hip extensors and the biceps femoris have to contract very strongly (see fig. 5.5, overleaf).

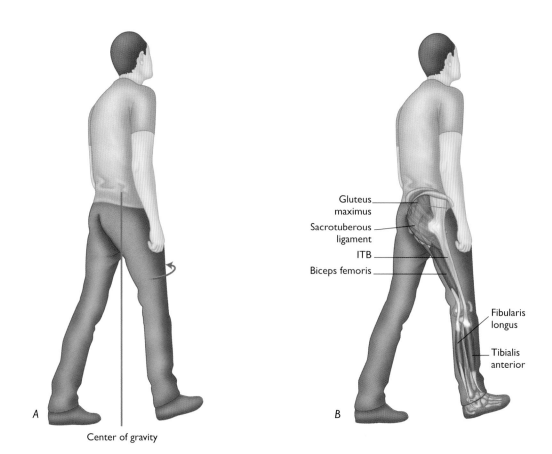

Gluteus maximus

Sacrotuberous ligament

ITB

Biceps femoris

Fibularis longus

Tibialis anterior

A

B

Center of gravity

Figure 5.5. A, In this position, with the hip flexed and the center of gravity behind the point of support, there will have to be a strong contraction within the hip extensors to prevent the body from falling. The biceps femoris is tensioned during the swing phase, prior to heel strike, by the hip flexion and by the supination of the foot, which tensions the myofascia of the fibularis longus. B, With eversion of the calcaneus and the chain of the medial rotations of the bones of the leg, there will be a consistent rotation from the hip to the sole of the foot.

The biceps femoris is an important part of the lower, posterior section of the Spiral Line and contracts with considerable force at heel strike (see fig. 5.5A). Thankfully, it is prepared for this, as it is stretched prior to impact by the dorsiflexion of the foot. Toward the latter stages of swing phase, the tibialis anterior draws the foot into dorsiflexion and some inversion, and this motion pulls on the fibularis longus, the tibialis anterior's antagonist in the dorsiflexion of the foot but also its neighbor in the continuity of the sling of the Spiral Line under the foot. This stretching of the fibularis longus brings the fibula downward and therefore lengthens the fascia of the biceps femoris (Vleeming et al. 2007). The biceps femoris is also being stretched by the flexion of the hip. Being "separated" from both ends like this helps the biceps femoris fascia to increase the efficiency of the hip extensors' activation. Activating from inside this tensed fascial encasement, the biceps femoris contracts at heel strike with more power, thereby doing less work and saving a few calories.

Some of the force of this contraction may be transmitted into the fibularis longus, pulling the fibula upward again and tensioning the fibularis longus from above as the tibialis anterior relaxes. This action will assist the sequence of pronation events in the foot, since the fibularis longus helps to draw the midtarsal bones into eversion, which unlocks the joints, opening the foot and allowing it to adapt to the ground surface.

The use of the gluteus maximus and biceps femoris gives us control at heel strike on two separate myofascial levels. The deeper hamstrings will bring the force to the sacrum and sacroiliac joints (see "The Pelvis" later in this chapter), and they will help decelerate knee flexion. The more superficial gluteus maximus allows the upper limb connection (see "Utilizing the Back Functional Line" below) and stretches to the front of the knee to control against knee flexion and internal rotation.

The anterior aspect of the line (tensor fascia lata and tibialis anterior) is passively tensioned with myofascial lengthening as the foot becomes less loaded and the lower limb passes into extension. This portion of the SPL is lengthened in a similar way to the Superficial Front Line as the pelvis moves over the foot rockers and the hip extends, but due to the more oblique fiber orientation, it assists with rotation as well as hip flexion.

If we look at the front of the leg (see fig. 5.5B), we can see a continual downward rotation pattern occurring as the foot pronates. This almost completely follows the classic Spiral Line as put forward by Myers, except for the connection from the iliotibial band to the ilium. Myers lists the tensor fascia lata as the continuity from the iliotibial band, but in terms of the function of the Spiral Line at this phase of gait, we have to redirect it to follow the line of force to the upper portion of gluteus maximus (see fig. 5.6, overleaf). This is not as much of a fudge when we realize that both the tensor fascia lata and the gluteus maximus are encased within the same fascial layer and both will be contracting to stabilize the pelvis in the frontal plane (we saw this earlier in the Lateral Line, see fig. 4.14, where the tensor fascia lata is loaded via hip adduction, as well as hip external rotation and knee flexion, at heel strike).

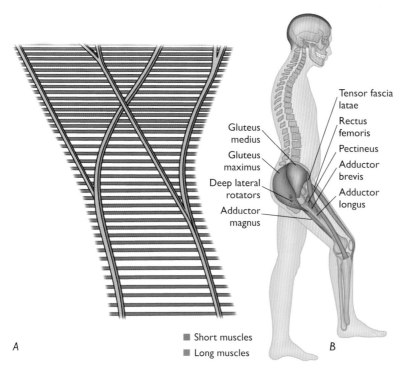

Gluteus medius

Gluteus maximus

Deep lateral rotators

Adductor magnus

Tensor fascia latae

Rectus femoris

Pectineus

Adductor brevis

Adductor longus

■ Short muscles
■ Long muscles

A

B

Figure 5.6. The greater trochanter is acting as what Myers calls a "switch" (or a "point" in the United Kingdom), the mechanism for changing tracks on a railway system. A, When the hip is flexed, the line of force travels posteriorly to the gluteus maximus; when extended, it goes to the tensor fascia lata.

Hydraulic Amplifier

The fascial sheets and the underlying muscle tissue can often cooperate to form a force amplification system, called the 'hydraulic amplifier effect,' as we saw in chapter 1 (see fig. 1.14b). Tensioning the fascial sheets increases the efficiency of the associated muscles, either in series or in parallel. This can be brought about in number of ways:

1. Tensioning of muscles embedded within the sheet. This is seen with tensor fascia lata and gluteus maximus, which are both encased within the fascia lata; the platysma within the fascia colli superficialis; and pectoralis minor contained within the clavipectoral fascia.

2. Muscles contracting deep to the fascial layer. For example, the contraction of the thigh muscles will tension the fascia lata from below, just as the erector spinae will tauten the posterior sheet of the thoracolumbar fascia.

3. The natural momentum of body movement can stretch and thereby elastically load the tissue. The swing of the arm will tension the thoracolumbar fascia; the swing of the leg will tension the epimysia of the hip extensors.

All three of these mechanisms can be and often are combined in functional movement. It is estimated that the hydraulic amplifier can increase efficiency of muscular work by up to 30 percent (DeRosa and Porterfield 2007) and so it is clearly a mechanism one wants to make full use of. When it is disrupted, such as by a fasciotomy, approximately 12 percent to 16 percent of efficiency can be lost (Gracovetsky 2008).

As the pelvis moves over the planted foot, the line of force will move from the gluteus maximus to the tensor fascia lata, or from the extensor to the flexor (see fig. 5.6), bringing us back to the true Spiral Line as outlined by Myers. Gluteus maximus contraction at heel strike is well established to be related to control of the knee, and failure to slow the internal rotation and frontal plane motion of the joint is often related to overpronation of the foot or to muscle weakness (Ireland et al. 2003; Powers et al. 2003). The relationship of the hip joint to the inside of the foot is therefore well established, and the line of force can be clearly observed—especially when it is exaggerated, such as in landing after a jump or changing direction while running (see fig. 5.7). A weak gluteus maximus is often blamed, but this is not necessarily the case. We regularly load muscles in two planes and then have to control the movement in the third; if insufficient loading occurs in one of the other planes, we lose the advantage for decelerating the third. Therefore, when looking at a possibly weak gluteus maximus, we need to check if the hip is adducting enough (to stretch it frontally) and flexing enough (to stretch it sagittally) so that it needs less contraction to control the transverse lengthening.

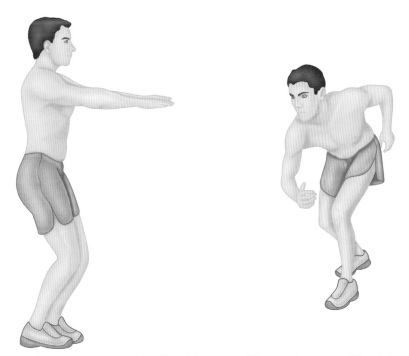

Figure 5.7. In other functional positions, we can see the effect of the increased force used in jumping (A) and changing direction (B). In either movement, weak gluteals can lead to lack of control of the valgus force at the knee and stress the medial collateral ligament or the lateral menisci. Alternatively, too much pronation of the bones of the foot can force the knee into a similar pattern, because of the mortise-and-tenon relationship of the tibia to the talus.

Utilizing the Back Functional Line—Connecting the Upper to the Lower Limb

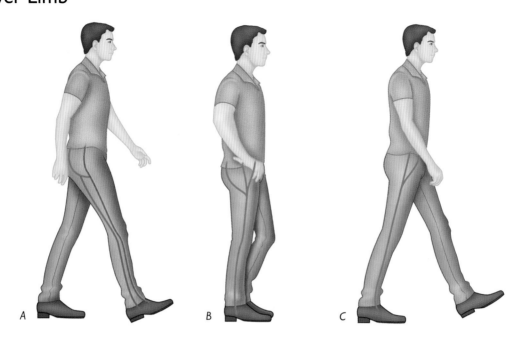

Figure 5.8. At the point of contact, there has to be a strong contraction in the extensors as well as the abductors. The extensors are pre-stretched by the hip flexion, the abductors by the lateral shift of the pelvis, creating the adduction of the hip, we saw in chapter 4. The opposite shoulder girdle adds support to the extended lower limb via the latissimus dorsi to the supporting gluteus maximus and down the front of the leg with the iliotibial band and tibialis anterior. The gluteus maximus is therefore being pre-stretched by opposite shoulder movement as well as by the hip flexion and adduction. All of this increases the body's potential efficiency through elastic recoil. As the pelvis moves over the planted foot, the line of force from the body's center of gravity moves from behind (A) to in line (B) and finally in front (C) of the point of support. This moves the need for contraction through the so-called deltoid of the hip (gluteus maximus, gluteus medius, and tensor fascia lata).

The gluteus maximus is also strongly connected to the latissimus dorsi on the opposite side of the body, and this relationship is renowned for its ability to increase stability. This connection has been thoroughly investigated by Vleeming (posterior sling), Zorn ('swingwalker'), as well as by Myers (Back Functional Line). This functional sling gives us a connection from the inside of the foot at heel strike (tibialis anterior) all the way to the opposite humerus (latissimus dorsi), both of which should be traveling in opposing directions. The first metatarsal—the attachment of tibialis anterior—will be heading for the floor, while the opposite arm is swinging forward and into a little external rotation, distally tensioning both ends of this adapted Spiral Line. This creates a long diagonal sling passing around the back of the flexed hip (via the thoracolumbar fascia, with gluteus maximus and latissimus attaching to it), which can then catapult the pelvis forward (see fig. 5.8a, and, for more information on the role of the thoracolumbar fascia/gluteus maximus link for energy saving, visit Adjo Zorn's site: www.swingwalker.net).

Once the pelvis has moved in front of the supporting foot, the line of force then engages through the tensor fascia lata (although it is a medial rotator of the thigh, it will be stretched and opened by the hip extension) and, through the continuity of the tibialis anterior, it will help lift the medial arch and will bring the femur, tibia and fibula, and the first metatarsal into a lateral rotation (see fig. 5.9).

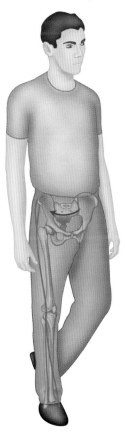

Figure 5.9. Once the pelvis moves in front of the foot, the hip is in extension and therefore begins to lengthen the tensor fascia lata. This engagement allows the anterior portion of the Spiral Line to assist with laterally rotating the lower limb, especially the foot, by helping lift the medial longitudinal arch to reengage the midtarsal joints.

Exercise 5.1. You can feel the relationship between the feet and the pelvis when standing comfortably with feet approximately hip-width apart and slowly tilting the pelvis anteriorly and posteriorly. In an anterior tilt, you may feel the knees overextend and medially rotate and the medial arch of the foot lower. With a posterior tilt you should feel the knees soften and laterally rotate and the medially arches lift.

The Potential Role of the Proprioceptors

Electromyography (EMG) readings of the hip extensors show that most of these muscles begin to contract prior to heel strike. The biceps femoris and semimembranosus start to contract as early as midswing (see fig. 5.10, overleaf), which could be due to the need for knee flexion, although knee flexion will occur naturally in response to gravity and doesn't require muscle force. The adductor magnus, gluteus maximus, and gluteus medius also begin to fire before contact is made with the ground. These early contractions are better explained, however, by the need to slow the forward swing of the leg, and they serve to prepare the fascial tissue for the loading that will occur at heel strike, thereby increasing the efficiency of the muscular contractions through pre-tension of the myofascial tissue.

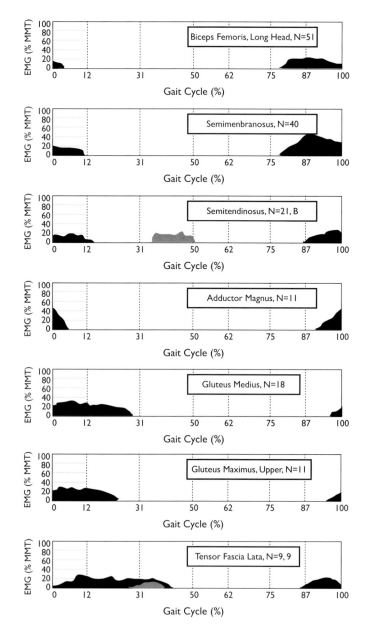

Figure 5.10.The charts showing percentage of maximum manual muscle test (MMT) and the phase of gait at which each muscle is active.We can clearly see that the hip extensors are firing before they are required to accept the weight of the body, from Mid-Swing (MSw) to Terminal Swing (TSw), and then following through to give their support in Initial Contact (IC, i.e., heel strike) and into Mid-Stance (MSt).Adapted from Perry and Burnfield 2010.

It seems logical that this anticipation is signaled via the lengthening of the fascia, stimulating the appropriate receptors as the thigh comes forward into hip flexion. The tone in the extensors and abductors allows for the immediate absorption of the natural "give" in the tissue around the joints, negating the need to quickly decelerate the movement, as would be necessary if the muscles were totally quiescent on landing.

After heel strike, the anterior portion of the Spiral Line lengthens very rapidly because of the eversion of the foot, and, remembering the work of Huijing (discussed in chapter 1), we can imagine the dispersal of mechanical information that will happen in response to this (see fig. 5.11). If this type of movement in the tissue is monitored by the proprioceptors (and research suggests that it is), it again seems reasonable to assume that this movement is what stimulates local muscle fibers.

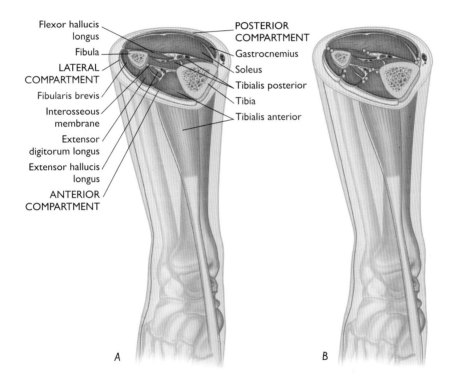

Figure 5.11. A, A change in tension, due to the ground reaction force and the downward pull of gravity, will send the force of the adjustment into the surrounding tissue, not only into the tibialis anterior. Presumably the tissue will be receiving signals from many other sources and then, on recognizing patterns, can create the necessary response in the muscle tone. B, Most of the proprioceptors are located in or around the septal divisions, which are the main borders between the muscles. The proprioceptors sense the variations in tension and shearing forces. Essentially, these areas are experiencing the most relative change in their relative biomechanics and so it makes sense to place the mechanoreceptors along these interfaces.

The mechanisms for activating the appropriate contraction of the correct muscles are therefore occurring in both sections of the lower Spiral Line but at different phases of the gait cycle. During mid- to late swing phase, it is the posterior hip extensors that are turned on, and then once the foot is planted and the limb begins to rotate, the new vector will further stimulate gluteus maximus as well as tibialis anterior. In both cases, the muscles are activated by the lengthening of their myofascia. The momentum of the leg swing stimulates the hip extensors, and the folding of the joints following the initial contact with the ground turns on the tibialis anterior and gluteus maximus.

The EMG readings of the anterior Spiral Line show an alternation between the active portions of the gait cycle, during which force must be carried or absorbed and work is performed by the muscle tissue to resist GRF or build momentum, and a more passive phase, during which the correction of position or initiation of an action is made by the fibrous elements, preferably through elastic energy. Both the swing phase of the thigh and the correction of the medial longitudinal arch occur when the tensor fascia lata and the tibialis anterior are electrically quiet, indicating a greater possibility of fascial involvement (see fig. 5.12).

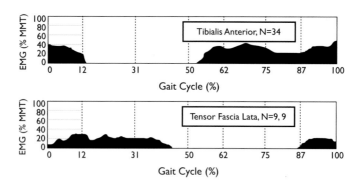

Figure 5.12. The EMG readings show the tibialis anterior as being electrically active from pre-swing (PS) through to loading response (LR). Presumably, it is stimulated during the swing phase by the weight of the foot loading the fascial tissue. The proprioceptors are stimulated and signal the muscle to lift the foot during the swing—to keep it clear of the ground—and then the muscle is quickly unloaded after receiving the forces of the body weight and momentum. Tensor fascia lata, as an abductor, is active through almost all of the stance phase, but it trails off before the leg swing occurs. This appears to indicate a passive mechanism for the hip flexion, as would be suggested by the fascial line and its recoil ability (and as felt in exercise 3.1). Adapted from Perry and Burnfield 2010.

THE UPPER BODY

As the Spiral Line travels up away from the anterior superior iliac spine (ASIS), the tissue of the tensor fascia lata continues into that of the abdominals. The continuity of the direction of force takes us to the internal obliques and then to the external obliques on the opposite side of the body. From the external obliques the line continues with the serratus anterior, which Myers has clearly shown to be myofascially continuous with the rhomboids. From there we cross the midline again to the splenius capitis to reach the head (see fig. 5.1).

We connected the rib cage and ilia with the Lateral Line, but those connections through the abdominals were ipsilateral and slightly more vertical. With the Spiral Line forces, we have to follow a diagonal line to the opposite-side rib cage, which leads into the upper attachments of the external obliques. These attachments are superficial to the myofascial level of the intercostals, which are deeper in the body and follow the "core" or "fish body"; instead, the obliques will lead us to the shoulder girdles via the serratus anterior.

The organization of the obliques and serratus anterior takes the tissue from being anchored on the trunk to being part of the shoulder girdle (Myers's "rhomboid-serratus muscle"). The line then returns to the trunk at the spinous processes to meet the splenius capitis and cervicis. This allows the shoulder girdles and the trunk to rotate independently of each other, contributing to our contralateral arm/leg swing.

We can see this arrangement when we look at the body from the top (see fig. 5.13, overleaf). The difference between the Lateral and Spiral Line obliques is that the former takes the rotation into the pliable rib cage, while the latter utilizes the opposite shoulder girdle, and thereby brings the arm movement and momentum into the equation for the counterrotation.

This organization in the tissue gives us three layers of rotation. The deepest is the rotation of the spine created by the Superficial Front and Back Lines, which turn the pelvis and therefore the sacrum. A middle layer of force is carried by the ipsilateral obliques of the Lateral Line to the rib cage. The most superficial—and the counterrotation to the others—is carried via the uppermost section of the Spiral Line (rhomboids and splenii). This counterrotation creates an external "balance spring" to the others. During relaxed walking, it seems to simply dissipate the rotational forces prior to reaching the head, while during vigorous walking, it is more actively engaged (whether held more stiffly or through concentric/eccentric contraction) and contributes a stronger counterrotation (see also "Spinal Engine" later in this chapter).

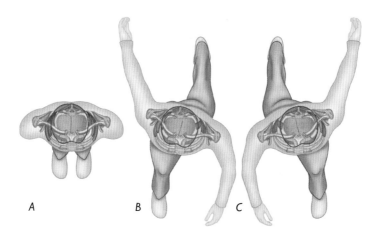

Figure 5.13. The upper portion of the Spiral Line gives us an axial-to-appendicular-to-axial link in the skeleton (A), which allows one to rotate independently of the other (B). However, this portion of the Spiral Line cannot be consistently short or long through its entirety: when the portion inferior to the medial border of the scapula is short (B), the superior portion will be long, and vice versa (C).

Our arm swing is contralateral to the swing of the lower limbs—when one arm is back, the leg on the opposite side will also be back. As we saw above, the lower portion of the Spiral Line (from the tensor fascia lata downward) passively assists the leg swing through fascial recoil. This may also be assisted by the upper Spiral Line, due to the shoulder being back and the pelvis dropping and rotating away from the rib cage on the opposite side (see fig. 5.14).

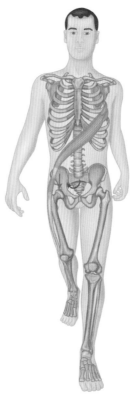

Figure 5.14. As the arm swings back, it helps to fascially engage the whole of the anterior Spiral Line from the medial border of one scapula to the opposite first metatarsal. The tension of the myofascia of the Spiral Line is enhanced by the pelvis shifting to the opposite side, adducting and rotating. Each of these movements increases the distance from the scapula to the opposite anterior superior iliac spine. We will see this contralateral pattern again later, as part of the Front Functional Lines.

As we see in figure 5.13, when the right leg is extended, the pelvis—and therefore the spine—rotates to the right. The shoulder girdle will be forward on the right, and if we look at the posterior portion of the upper Spiral Line (see fig. 5.14), we can clearly see that the forward momentum of the right shoulder creates a stretch on the spinous processes of the mid- and upper thoracic spine. This may help produce the counterrotation of the spine, or at least reduce the rotation created in the pelvis before it reaches the head.

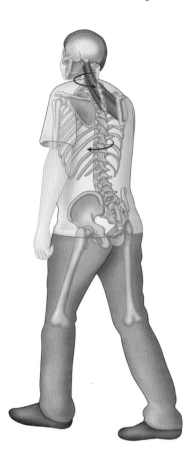

Figure 5.15. As the arm swings forward, it creates a pull through the rhomboids and the splenius, which may help reduce the spinal rotation coming from the pelvis.

There is an alternating pattern of stretch in the upper Spiral Line: as the tissue on the front of the trunk is stretched on one side by the posterior swing of the arm, the tissue on the back of the other side is shortened (see fig. 5.14 and 5.15). This is allowed by the paradoxical relationship of the rhomboid-serratus sling, the two sides of which cannot be short (or long) at the same time.

THE PELVIS

When the feet are at the extremes of the gait cycle—heel strike and push-off—the ilia will be relatively posteriorly and anteriorly tilted, respectively (see fig. 5.16). We saw this as part of the effect of the Superficial Back and Front Lines. This position will be corrected naturally through the weight acceptance, stance, and swing phase movements by the SBL and SFL. The Spiral Line appears to influence the sacroiliac joint and the three-dimensional movement through this complex in healthy walking.

If we heel strike with the right foot, the right ilium will be posteriorly tilted (you can feel this on yourself if you are not familiar with it). The ilium moves farther and faster than the sacrum, so the sacrum will be anteriorly titled relative to the ilium on the right side. This relationship is known as *nutation* (see fig. 5.16).

As we heel strike on the right, we will be preparing for push-off on the left, and this will then create the opposite tilts of the ilium and sacrum on the left side, thereby causing a relative posterior tilt or "counter-nutation" of the sacrum at the left sacroiliac joint.[1]

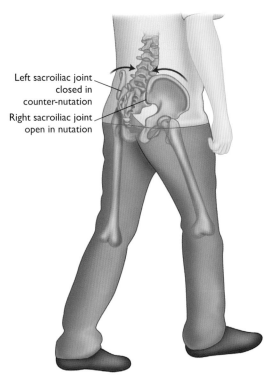

Left sacroiliac joint
closed in
counter-nutation

Right sacroiliac joint
open in nutation

Figure 5.16. When the heel strikes, the femur will be posteriorly tilted, drawing the ilium with it, while the reverse relationship will be occurring on the opposite side. This creates a nutation on the side of heel strike and a counter-nutation on the other.

1 The use of counter-nutation at the sacroiliac joint in function is debatable, as some argue that the sacroiliac joints are always nutated in weight bearing. I use it here to describe the joint's position relative to the opposite side, not the actual position at the joint.

The sacrum sits in the pelvis like a hammock, with the dorsal sacroiliac ligaments supporting it like ropes from the trees of the ilia (see fig. 5.17A). The anterior tilt of the human pelvis is in contrast to the ape's, whose pelvis sits almost parallel to the spine. The evolution of the human pelvis appears to provide the sacroiliac joints with the ability to reduce the forces coming from the lower limbs before those forces reach the spine. The suspension arrangement of the sacroiliac joints and their nutation/counter-nutation movements create a natural shock absorber that tolerates relative motion in all three planes of movement.

Restriction in the sacroiliac joints transfers more movement from the ilia to the sacrum and spine. If the ligaments are unable to allow movement, the sacrum will be forced to follow movement of the ilia, and then the L5 vertebra will be forced to follow the sacrum. The client, however, may compensate with less lower limb movement, especially limiting their hip flexion and extension, to reduce the tilting of the ilia.

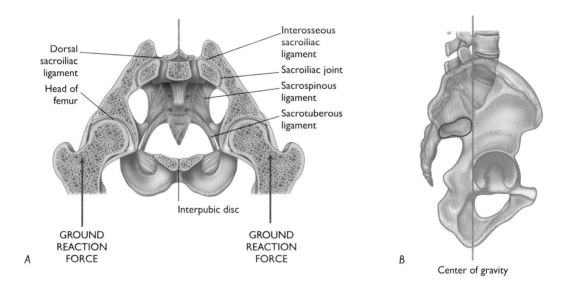

Figure 5.17. With the cross section in the frontal plane (A), we can see how the sacrum is suspended from the ilia. This arrangement allows each of the three bones to move relative to the others. If we imagine the sacrum in the middle as a hammock and the dorsal sacroiliac ligaments as the ropes, the ilia are therefore like the supporting trees (as seen above in 5.16). The arrangement is enhanced by the almost horizontal orientation of the sacrum, which increases slightly when in standing.

However, the nutation and counter-nutation movements of the pelvis are very small and must be contained. Both the Spiral and the Superficial Back Lines blend into the sacrotuberous ligament via the hamstrings, and one of that ligament's many functions is to control the nutation of the sacrum.

In recently published articles, Jap van Der Waal, a Dutch anatomist, has revisited work from his 1988 doctoral thesis and promoted the concept of "dynaments" (his suggested contraction of "dynamic ligament"). In his model, which is based on many dissections, he suggests that we should reconsider the idea that ligaments are primarily passive supporting structures. Instead, he shows that most ligaments actually lie in series with the contractile tissue (i.e., they are continuous with the muscle) and are therefore tensioned by it. In the case of the Spiral Line, we should consider the sacrotuberous ligament as an extended tendon of the hamstrings—of the biceps femoris in particular (Willard, in Vleeming et al. 2007). The implication of this is that the sacrotuberous ligament has an active, functional role—it encourages the return of the sacrum from a nutated position (see fig. 5.18). This is a simple reversal of roles: the passive job of the ligaments (the prevention of movement) is altered by the incorporation of an active contraction, making them an extension of the muscular elements (they lie "in series" with the muscle) and thereby involved in the creation of movement.

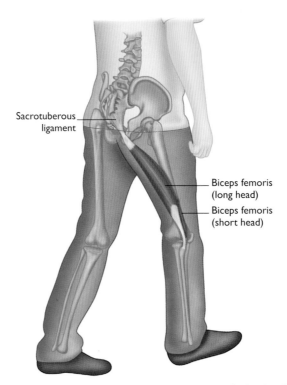

Sacrotuberous ligament

Biceps femoris (long head)

Biceps femoris (short head)

Figure 5.18. The contraction of the hamstrings on heel strike and the loading to prevent further hip flexion creates tension that must be carried through onto the sacrotuberous ligament. This contraction prevents additional nutation of the sacroiliac joint and may also help its return to a neutral position.

On the opposite side of the sacrum, the long dorsal sacroiliac ligament "officially" helps prevent counter-nutation. The long dorsal sacroiliac ligament is connected to the erector spinae and somewhat to the multifidi. Vleeming and Stoeckart found that tractioning the erectors led to an increase in tension in this ligament (Vleeming et al. 2007) and so if we rethink this ligament as being a "dynament" it will create nutation on contraction of the low back extensors.

Follow the exercise below and you will feel a contralateral relationship between the hamstrings and the erectors at the point of heel strike (multifidi and the erectors will activate on both sides of the spine but more so on the "swing side"). By following the

Spiral Line to the opposite side of the sacrum via this functional sling of sacrotuberous to long dorsal sacroiliac ligament we now have an oblique tensioning of support and correction for the action of the SIJs (see fig. 5.18).

Exercise 5.2: Place your right hand on your right hamstrings and the back of your left hand across the erector spinae of your low back and take a few steps. What do you feel at the point of heel strike on the right?

Hopefully you feel a strong tensioning of the hamstrings on the right and of the erector spinae on the left.

Repeat exercise 3.3 to feel the opposing motions of the ilia in walking (the ilium on the side of heel strike should be tilting back). Imagine what is happening to the sacroiliac joint inside. As the ilium tilts back, it moves farther than the sacrum, making it "nutate" relative to the position of the sacrum.

Feel—and then picture—what is happening on the extended limb: the ilium is anteriorly tilting and the sacroiliac joint is counter-nutating. Imagine a line between the sacrotuberous ligament and the posterior superior iliac spine and feel this as the axis of correction. As you step, can you internally sense that line becoming taut to help correct the torsion that occurs in the sacroiliac joint?

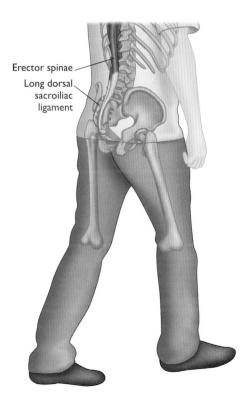

Figure 5.19. With the long dorsal sacroiliac ligament now in place, you can see the axis that may help with the three-dimensional movement of the sacrum in the sacroiliac joint.

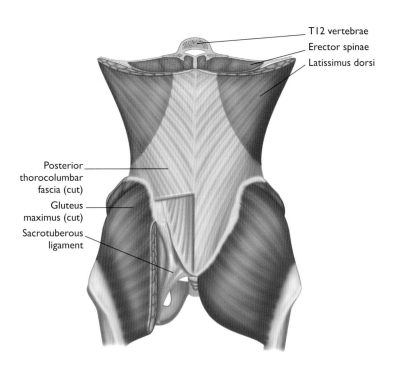

Figure 5.20. The contraction of the erectors deep to the tensioned thoracolumbar fascia will also assist with the "hydraulic amplification" in this segment.

Note: While both the Superficial Back Line and the Spiral Line overlap by coming through the hamstrings (or part of them) to the sacrotuberous ligament, the idea of the Spiral Line and not the Superficial Back Line passing to the opposite side is a conceptual rather than actual differentiation. The Superficial Back Line refers more to movements in the sagittal plane (such as many of the forward and backward bends used in Pilates and yoga), while the Spiral Line refers to the rotations and oblique angles that will help us negotiate the transverse plane adaptations that occur in rotatory movement patterns.

This returns us to one of the Anatomy Trains principles, which dictates we must follow the line of pull (or tension) in the tissue. This will clearly be affected by position and mechanics of the action occurring across the joints at any one time, and this is what leads to the need to use the switch at the greater trochanter to adjust the line of the SPL to follow the gluteus maximus.

REDUCING THE SPIRAL

As we noted above, the Spiral Line travels from tissue levels that are relatively superficial to ones that are deep. Starting[2] at the splenius capitis and cervicis, it wraps around and down the body and legs, eventually coming back up the body to the sacrotuberous ligament and then back up to the head with the opposite erector spinae, under the bandages of the splenii (see fig. 5.21). As it does so, it also gradually reduces its oblique angle and becomes almost vertical along the erector spinae.

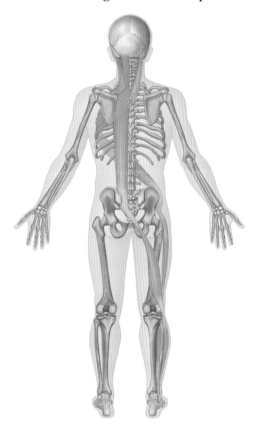

Figure 5.21. Starting from the splenii, the Spiral Line begins superficially, near the surface of the body, and during its tour of the body, it gradually sinks toward the body's interior, until it reaches the deeper layer of the erectors for its return to the head. Its momentum for rotation is also reducing as it progresses, especially up the posterior aspect, where it is essentially vertical.

This may be part of the function of the SPL: not only to create and maintain the contralateral rotations from the upper girdles through the pelvis to the lower limbs, but also to act as a damper for the sacroiliac joints and especially for the spine against those rotations. This is particularly evident when we look at the very upper portion (the splenius/rhomboids sling), which, in function, acts in reverse to the tissue joining the upper girdle to the opposite anterior superior iliac spine. In this way, the SPL may function more as described by Dart, who saw the rotational relationships of the oblique tissues in joining the pelvic and shoulder girdles (1996, fig 5.22, see overleaf).

2 None of the Anatomy Trains lines 'starts' anywhere; any sequencing of the myofascial elements is purely for convenience of description.

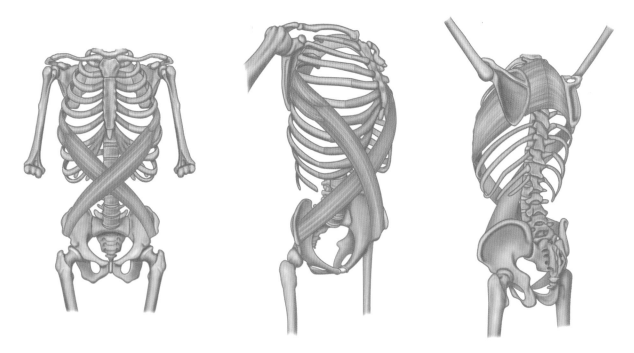

Figure 5.22. This figure shows the spiral relationship through the torso from one anterior superior iliac spine through the shoulder girdles to the opposite one. This is a contrast to Myers's Spiral Line, which includes the lower limbs and assists with its rotational patterns.

The Spinal Engine

One does not need legs to be a nomad.
—Zygmunt Bauman

Gracovetsky posits, in his Spinal Engine Theory, that the three sections of the spine function cooperatively during the rotations of walking (see fig. 5.23). The pelvis and lumbars are coupled together in rotation, as discussed earlier in the SFL and SBL in chapter 3 (see also fig. 5.23): when the lower limbs are in flexion and extension the pelvis rotates to accommodate the length of the stride. The inability of the lumbars to absorb the rotation (due to their limitations in the transverse plane, see fig. 5.24) sends the rotational forces up to the thoracics, which, due to the counterrotation of the shoulder girdles, creates fascial tensioning and wind-up in the rotatores and multifidi. According to Gracovetsky, these two rotations should ideally meet somewhere around T8 and act somewhat like a watch spring. The natural momentum of the rotation serves to tension the tissues, which then recoil into the reverse rotation. Using spinal facet and oblique tissue alignment, Gracovetsky argues that we do not require the lower limbs for movement, the two rotations from the upper body are enough to propel us forward.

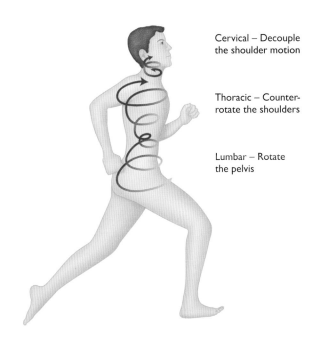

Cervical – Decouple
the shoulder motion

Thoracic – Counter-
rotate the shoulders

Lumbar – Rotate
the pelvis

Figure 5.23. The three spinal sections, according to Gracovetsky, contribute to the transverse motion of gait. The lumbars move with the pelvis, and the thoracics counterrotate, because of the shoulder girdle, leading to tensioning in the oblique muscles of the spine. The cervical region is uncoupled from the rest of the spine, both in its facet arrangement and through the arrangement of the soft tissue, which allows it to maintain the forward gaze of the head. Adapted from Gracovetsky 2008.

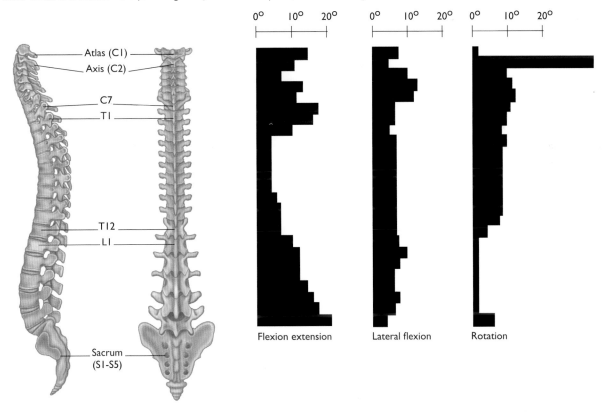

Figure 5.24. Because of the lack of rotation in the lumbars, their ability to absorb transverse plane movement is limited. The pelvic rotation caused by the reach of the forward leg therefore transfers into the thoracic vertebrae, as described in chapter 4, as it is carried upward via the X of the obliques in the Lateral Line. The facets of the thoracic vertebrae are aligned a little more in the frontal plane and thereby allow more rotation. The counterrotation of the upper girdle then encourages a meeting of these opposing rotations around the level of T8, producing a fascial recoil in the transverse plane. Adapted from Middleditch and Oliver 2005.

The forward swing of the arm tensions the rhomboids and the splenii portion of the Spiral Line, which helps to rotate the upper thoracic spine and the head in the opposite direction from that of the lumbars and lower thoracics. This counterrotation of the spine and rib cage neutralizes the rotation of the lower body, which helps to stabilize the head in the transverse plane.

The Spiral Line therefore adds a mechanism to correct the torsion of the pelvis via the two sacral ligaments, as well as helping create Gracovetsky's "Spinal Engine" mechanism. It manages this because of its unique pattern of gradually sinking into a deeper, more interior layer of the body. Starting superficially on the head with the splenius capitis, it wraps around the body with the rhomboid-serratus muscle and the obliques to the tensor fascia lata and iliotibial band—or, using the Back Functional Line, it can also "begin" at the arm, with the latissimus dorsi, and stretch from the lats and gluteus maximus and thence into the iliotibial band. From the iliotibial band, the SPL tracks to the sacrotuberous ligament via the tibialis anterior, fibularis longus, and biceps femoris, and eventually goes to the erector spinae, truly axial muscles.

The Spiral Line allows us to use the superficial tissue associated with the cervical spine and the shoulder girdles to add a corrective outer spring to our watch mechanism. (As an aside, this is exactly how Robert Hooke developed greater accuracy for his watch spring. He found that a second spring compensated for the changes in tension of the first spring as it unwound.) The tissue of the Lateral Line brings the rotation of the pelvis into the rib cage, and then the more superficial Spiral Line tissue uses the counterrotation of the shoulders to add opposing transverse forces into the equation, producing greater efficiency for the transverse plane movement and taking advantage of the spinal mechanics.

The Spiral Line is involved with nearly all the movements necessary for walking—foot pronation and its correction to supination, the rotations and flexions and extensions of the lower limbs, the movement at the sacrum and into the spine, the rotation of the trunk and counterrotations of the shoulder girdles—all of which help to keep the head steady. However, as we shall see in the next chapter, to function efficiently, the Spiral Line requires feedback and support from the Deep Front Line in order to balance the trunk on top of the legs.

SUMMARY

1. Pre-tension of the hip extensors is created by the deceleration of hip flexion during swing phase and is assisted by ankle dorsiflexion. The tibialis anterior is contracted to lift the foot and, via the fibularis longus, draws down on the head of the fibula to further tension the biceps femoris, thereby pulling it from both ends.

2. At heel strike, the Spiral Line uses the switch of the greater trochanter to engage the Back Functional Line (the gluteus maximus and latissimus dorsi) to help control and decelerate the pronation pattern created by the offset talus on the calcaneus.

3. The deeper posterior section of the SPL assists with the correction of the sacroiliac joints, using the continuity of the biceps femoris and sacrotuberous ligament to produce counter-nutation, and using the opposite erector spinae and long dorsal sacroiliac ligament to nutate the sacrum on the side of the extended leg.

4. As the body progresses through weight acceptance toward push-off, the greater trochanter switch turns to the tensor fascia lata and the oblique line to the opposite shoulder girdle. This long anterior line can be engaged to help with hip flexion (tensor fascia lata / iliotibial band, tibialis anterior) and to support the supination of the foot prior to the propulsion.

5. The posterior X of the upper Spiral Lines creates the counterrotation in the upper thoracic spine to oppose the rotation driven from the pelvis, which helps stabilize the head. On one side of the body, as the anterior part of the upper SPL assists movement of the lower limb, the posterior portion (rhomboids and splenii) on that side will be shorter—and the reverse will be true on the other side of the body. This crossover in tension between the portions of the lines creates the counterrotation necessary for Gracovetsky's "Spinal Engine" and allows the skull to remain straight.

6. The superficial aspects of the SPL help more with the overall kinetic forces, while the deeper sections reduce the rotational torques and ease the joint mechanics.

ESSENTIAL EVENTS

Pronation/Supination

The talar joint is responsible for the sagittal plane movements, while the subtalar (talocalcaneal joint) creates inversion and eversion. We have to put them in context with the even-longer-named talocalcaneonavicular joint (a rounded ball-and-socket type joint) and the calcaneocuboidal joint (a gliding joint). It is the latter two that produce the movements of supination and pronation, which lock and unlock the midtarsal joints respectively.

The bones of the client's feet should be able to open and adapt on heel strike and then need to reengage in preparation for push-off. This can be assessed somewhat during gait, but it will be easier to see by having the client move his or her knee over the medial and lateral aspects of the foot. These actions will create internal and external rotation of the talus to pronate and supinate the foot (see fig. 5.25). Standing relaxed and using one leg at a time removes any other possible restriction that may interfere with the test.

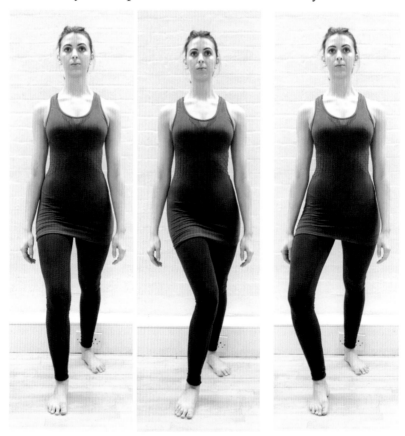

Figure 5.25. In this first position the client is relaxed and simply moves the knee medially and laterally, which should create pronation and supination, respectively. To assess this ability in gait see fig. 5.26.

Once that has been done, in the second stage of the test the client stands in a more gait-like position to mimic the tissue relationships (see fig. 5.26).

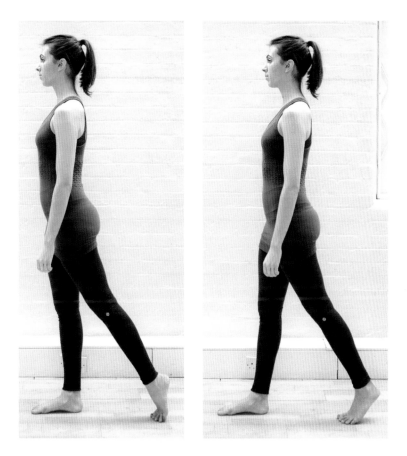

Figure 5.26. Using a split stance, transfer the body weight onto the forward foot to assess for pronation of the front foot.

Sacroiliac Joint Mobility

For the pelvis to torsion correctly, with the ilia traveling in opposite directions, the sacroiliac joints must be mobile. A restriction on one side could lead to overextension on the other side, as well as uneven loading into the spine.

There are many tests to assess the sacroiliac joints, but they often give contradictory results, so it is best to assess the joints in the context of a normal gait, by feeling for the torsion as the client either walks or transfers his or her body weight forward and back while standing in a position similar to that used in figure 5.26.

Shoulder Girdle Counter Swing

Various studies have shown that the arm swing adds little to the efficiency of the gait. This seems to be a case of "science" saying one thing and experience another. The quote of Nicholson, which helps open chapter 1 ("walking while nursing an injured arm in a cast throws off your balance and distorts your geometry of the walking body, creating various tensions and asymmetries that in themselves create further pain") attests to the idea that—while not essential to walking—our arms do add a certain *je ne sais quoi*. Try walking at speed without swinging your arms, and you will feel their loss—or, as Nicholson did, try walking with one arm in a heavy cast.

Imbalances in arm swing can be clues to further weaknesses in the system. Too much swing, especially on one side, can indicate weak gluteals, as the latissimus dorsi tries to compensate through the Back Functional Line. Insufficient swing (or lack of swing) may be due to shortness in this line, that is, if the Back Functional line is short and one tries to use a longer arm swing, it could encourage too much rotation of the opposite femur.

An overall increase in swing can indicate a lack of rotation through the thoracic cage, because increased swing can compensate for such immobilization.

Arm swing can be dependent on the speed of movement, so assessing the client at varying paces can be useful. With increased speed, expect an increased range of arm swing.

6 Deep Front Line

OUR INNER SPRING

I raised me, as good walkers should, and bore
My body upright, though the thoughts in me
Remained bowed down and shrunken as before.
—Dante, *The Divine Comedy*

INTRODUCTION

The inner connection and blending of the myofascia and the visceral fascia that occurs through the Deep Front Line (DFL) may be one reason why a walk in the country on a beautiful spring day feels so much easier than a winter's trudge to work. Our human condition allows us many different moods, and most are reflected in our body use. It may be the center of our beings—the core—that makes the difference. For example, imagine your movement if you were to walk with a sense of depression or sadness. That internal deflation would rob something from the spring in your step.

Some of that loss may be due to a shorter stride, as discussed earlier, but much will also result from the lower muscle tone and loss of connection through the center of our bodies, the tissue which is referred to as the Deep Front Line (DFL). Unlike the Spiral Line, which crosses the body from left to right and right to left, the Deep Front Line fills the body's inner space.

Connecting the muscles of the jaw all the way to the soles of the feet via the neck and the chest, abdomen and pelvis, the DFL is often referred to as the "core." While this may be an overused and under-defined term, it does give a sense of the inner support that a toned and engaged Deep Front Line provides.[1] As we will see, the DFL is used at both heel strike (hip flexion) and push-off (hip extension). This occurs through the connections of the flexor and extensor adductors that stretch from the diaphragm and the pelvic floor to the feet.

---

[1] By calling the DFL 'engaged,' I do not intend to invoke the conventional 'core exercises' that deliberately contract the muscles but rather the mechanical engagement of the line that happens when appropriate movement allows the myofascia of the line to be stimulated.

THE INNER MECHANICS

In movement, the Deep Front Line (fig. 6.1) takes us in different directions using a number of "switches"—junctions—but in this case, unlike the Spiral Line, we can stay true to the original outline of this Anatomy Train. In the leg, the Deep Front Line (DFL) begins with the three muscles of the deep posterior compartment and then crosses the medial aspect of the knee and divides into the anterior and posterior adductors. The myofascial divergence above the knee creates the switch that allows this line to be active in both hip flexion and extension, with the adductors stretching anteriorly and posteriorly to the hip joint. From their respective attachments at the hip, they will lead us into the pelvic, abdominal, and thoracic cavities, and finally come to the head via the hyoid complex and the throat.

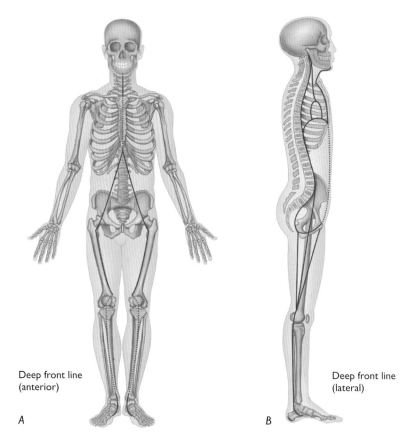

Deep front line
(anterior)

A

Deep front line
(lateral)

B

Figure 6.1. The Deep Front Line takes us on a journey through the center of the body. Often referred to as the "core," many see it as being responsible for our inner support, anterior (A) and lateral (B) views.

The Deep Front Line certainly incorporates much of the intimate myofascia associated with inner support and vitality. Its fascia surrounds our viscera, the sensitive organs of the body, and is closely associated with our emotional states and even our sexuality. Many factors are therefore involved in allowing this important line to play its diverse roles in movement. It requires balance with the more superficial myofascial lines, which must be free enough to allow the tensional forces to travel to the deeper tissue (see fig. 6.2). Conversely, issues from within the DFL, such as internal health (whether emotional or structural) can be reflected to the outside, often forcing the outer lines—the "sleeve" surrounding the DFL—to compensate for an impaired core.

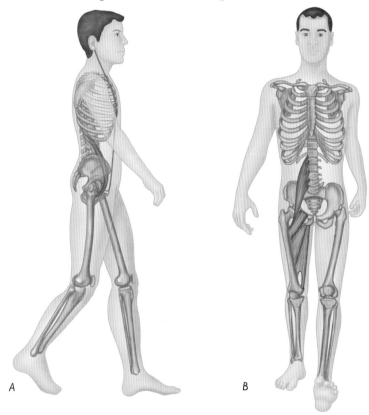

A   B

Figure 6.2. If the client is unable to fully lengthen the superficial tissue, in this case the rectus femoris of the SFL, it prevents the mechanical tensioning of the psoas in the sagittal plane. This can lead to overuse issues, or it may lead to a compensation pattern in which the client uses external hip rotation to enlist the adductors for hip flexion (B).

The ability to see and recognize these patterns is important, as they can happen anywhere in the body, through any of the other superficial lines, preventing the mechanical load reaching the Deep Front Line, which will inhibit the DFL's ability to assist with the desired movement. Easy and graceful movement occurs when the superficial and deep lines are able to work together, each doing their fair share of the work.

THE FOOT

The myofascia of the Deep Front Line is strongly associated with the support of the medial longitudinal arch and the midtarsal joints that make up the complex system within the foot. The tendons of the flexors hallucis and digitorum longus and tibialis posterior give us the final set of strings within a series of pulleys that work in concert to produce supination.

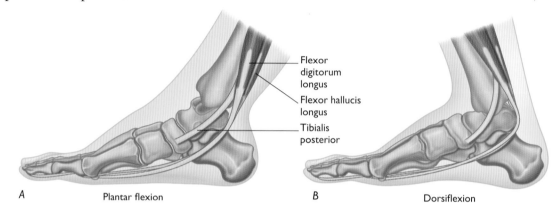

Flexor
digitorum
longus

Flexor hallucis
longus

Tibialis
posterior

A   Plantar flexion   B   Dorsiflexion

Figure 6.3. The three tendons of the deep posterior compartment all wrap around the back of the medial malleolus, which acts like a pulley—as the ankle dorsiflexes (B), the tendons will be tensioned, and they draw the bones of the foot together. It is almost like lacing your shoes: by pulling on the laces, you draw the sides of the shoe together, using the eyelets as the pulley. See also fig. 6.9.

Each of the tendons of the deep posterior compartment wraps around the medial malleolus and dives under the sole of the foot. Of these, the flexor hallucis longus is especially important, as it threads its way below the sustentaculum tali, the promontory of the calcaneus supporting the talus. These three tendons also play an important role in preparing the foot for push-off, by being tensioned in dorsiflexion, and may be an accessory part of the windlass mechanism mentioned in chapter 3 (see fig. 6.3).

The fascia from the deep posterior compartment carries us over the medial aspect of the knee and onto the femur. From here, the tissue continues with the adductors. When considering pelvic tilts and shifts, we may need to address the adductors, as they can affect the position of the pelvis. But in the function of walking, the adductors convey the tensional changes from the pelvis to the medial longitudinal arch.

ANTERIOR SEPTUM

If we follow the anterior portion of the adductors from the medial epicondyle (the adductor tubercle), the fascial compartment will bring us toward the lesser trochanter via the distal portions of the adductors longus and brevis and the pectineus. These muscles attach to the pubic ramus, but their septal fascia will merge with that of the iliacus and psoas, as their conjoined tendon crosses the front of the pelvis. This anterior line therefore joins the inside of the foot to the diaphragm via three paths: the psoas, the quadratus lumborum and iliacus, and the pectineus and psoas minor (see fig. 6.4).

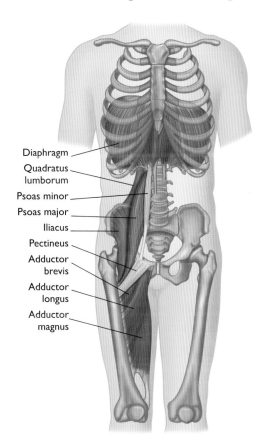

Diaphragm
Quadratus lumborum
Psoas minor
Psoas major
Iliacus
Pectineus
Adductor brevis
Adductor longus
Adductor magnus

Figure 6.4. Once the fascia of the anterior adductors reach the lesser trochanter, they continue to the diaphragm via three paths: the "express" of the psoas (red); the iliacus, which blends with the fascia of the quadratus lumborum (blue); and the pectineus, which leads to the psoas minor (yellow). These three continuities give us a strong association between the diaphragm and the upper thigh muscles that will be engaged during hip extension, especially when combined with internal rotation and abduction (as shown). This combination is the ideal position to engage through this fascial line at push-off.

POSTERIOR SEPTUM

If we return to the medial epicondyle, the posterior adductor septum will go to the ischiopubic ramus with the adductor magnus, which blends into the fascia of the obturator internus and, thereby, the pelvic floor. From the pelvic floor, the myofascial continuity continues to the head via the anterior longitudinal ligament or the deep aspect of the transversus abdominis, which blends with the abdominal and thoracic intracavity linings, leading us into the throat to reach the cranium (see fig. 6.5). As we will see later in this chapter, the tensioning of the posterior line in the thigh is important for "core" support at heel strike.

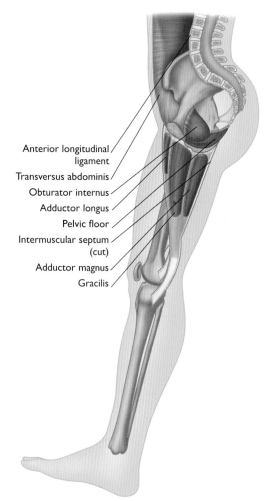

Anterior longitudinal ligament
Transversus abdominis
Obturator internus
Adductor longus
Pelvic floor
Intermuscular septum (cut)
Adductor magnus
Gracilis

Figure 6.5. The posterior septum will bring us along the adductor magnus to the ischiopubic ramus, blending into the obturator internus and from there to the pelvic floor. The continuity from the pelvic floor can also go in two directions—anteriorly, with the transversus abdominis, or along the front of the spine with the anterior longitudinal ligament. Both of these tracks will bring us to the cranium.

Much of the inner support for the head may come from the tissues of the Deep Front Line. If we continue the line from the back of the transversus abdominis, it brings us to the tissue on the back of the sternum and eventually upward to the infrahyoids and suprahyoids. Many of the deep anterior supporting muscles of the neck, such as the longus capitis and colli (see fig. 6.6), are a continuation of tissues ascending from the diaphragm, which we reached using the psoas and quadratus lumborum. Therefore, if the head is correctly placed on the top of the cervical spine and supported by the muscles ascending from the thoracic cage, in balance with the erectors, then the superficial tissues of the shoulder muscles should be free to perform their duties for the shoulders—if we are standing still. However, as we will see in the next chapter, once we begin to move, the head becomes a very heavy and potentially unstable unit on top of a slender pole of support. In function, therefore, the head requires the extra lines of tension coming from superficial tissues, especially those connecting it to the shoulders (see chapter 7).

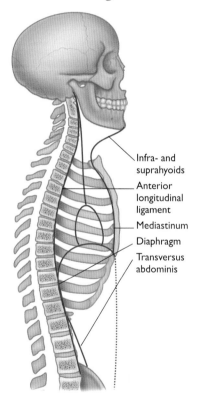

Figure 6.6. The Deep Front Line incorporates much of (if not all) our internal, visceral fascia. For our purposes, however, we follow the three main myofascial lines Myers describes to reach the front of the cranium—the hyoids leading to the muscles of the jaw, the muscles supporting the front of the neck and the anterior longitudinal ligament leading to the foramen magnum (2009).

DEEP FRONT LINE—PRONATION TO SUPINATION

In the preparation for push-off, the medial longitudinal arch should correct from pronation, allowing the midtarsal joints to reengage and create a more stable foot to push from. A number of mechanisms will be involved in this procedure, one through the bones and two via the soft tissue.

It is the action of the swing leg coming through into flexion that stimulates each of these mechanisms. As we saw in the Superficial Front and Back Lines (chapter 3), the swing leg causes a rotation of the pelvis to the opposite side, which rotates the supporting femur (the stance leg) laterally. This rotation will encourage the tibia and the fibula to rotate in the same direction. Held as it is in the mortise between the malleoli, the talus will also turn, lifting the calcaneus with it (as described in chapter 2).

This mechanism of the bones is supported by the soft tissue of the Spiral Line (chapter 5). Once the leg comes into extension, the line of tissue from the tensor fascia lata to the tibialis anterior will be pulled, thereby lifting the base of the first metatarsal, the distal part of the arch.

The third mechanism providing foot supination is the tensioning of the Deep Front Line, as mentioned above. Prior to push-off, the hip joint will be in extension, internal rotation, and abduction, ideal positions to load the psoas, iliacus, and anterior adductors. Also, the foot will be dorsiflexed and the knee extended. These positions create an engagement of the anterior DFL all the way from the neck to the inside of the foot, but especially from the diaphragm through the psoas (see exercise 6.1 and fig. 6.7).

Exercise 6.1. Step forward with one leg, keeping the heel of the back foot on the floor. Internally rotate your back leg slightly and then slowly bring your pelvis into a posterior tilt or experiment with bringing it forward and back slightly. Can you feel the arch lift slightly as you tilt back and/or as you bring the pelvis forward? Can you feel the connection from the front of the pelvis across the inside of the back of the knee to the medial arch? You may feel a stretch along the anterior septum of the thigh, the inside of the knee, or even along the medial aspect of the tibia, but wherever the sensation is, it will be somewhere along this strong fascial line of the anterior DFL.

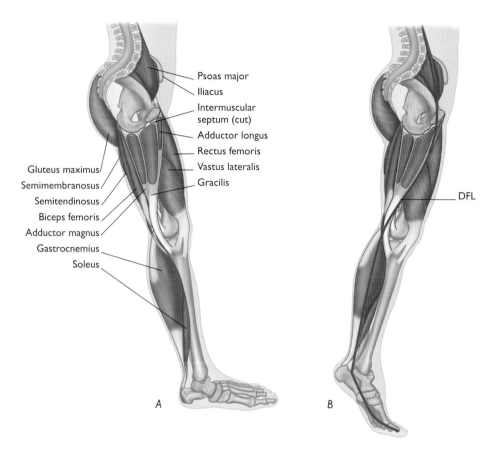

Psoas major
Iliacus
Intermuscular
septum (cut)
Adductor longus
Rectus femoris
Vastus lateralis
Gracilis

Gluteus maximus
Semimembranosus
Semitendinosus
Biceps femoris
Adductor magnus
Gastrocnemius
Soleus

DFL

A

B

Figure 6.7. A, Immediately after heel strike the anterior portion of the Deep Front Line adductors will be disengaged—due to hip and knee flexion—allowing the foot to pronate in response to the ground reaction force. B, As we come into hip extension and ankle dorsiflexion the line comes into a Z-shaped stretch as the tissue wraps around the pulleys of the front of the pubic ramus and the back of the medial malleolus.

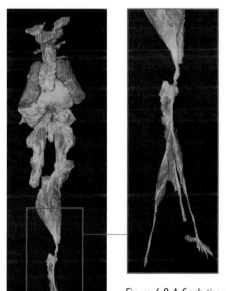

Figure 6.8. A fresh tissue dissection demonstrates the presence of this strong myofascial connection from the front of the pelvis to the inside of the foot. Note the strong tendinous element between the medial epicondyle, along the medial aspect of the knee joint to the popliteus and into the deep posterior compartment (shown in inset). Many people feel this section "pull" when doing exercise 6.1, and the orientation of the fibers shows that it is more involved with this vertical transfer of force from walking than with the oblique pull from the popliteus, with which it is continuous.

The Z-shaped stretch that is created in the DFL compliments the actions of the Lateral and Spiral Lines. The tissue of the tibialis anterior (of the Spiral Line) will be drawn up by the extension occurring at the hip and by the lateral rotation of the tibia to help lift the base of the first metatarsal. The fibularii longus and brevis (of the Lateral Line) will be tensioned by the dorsiflexion of the ankle, as they wrap around the lateral malleolus. The fibularis longus will meet and further support the tibialis anterior, combining their efforts to stabilize the mobile first ray (see fig. 6.9).

As the ankle dorsiflexes, the fibularis brevis will draw the fifth metatarsal into the cuboid to provide lateral stability, but it—and its longer compatriot—must be in balance with the medial tissues of the DFL and allow the ankle to dorsiflex evenly. A common pattern is for the lateral band of the plantar fascia or the fibularis tendons to be short, which causes them to hold the foot in a lateral rotation. This prevents the corrective supination of the foot that should occur in order to engage the midtarsal joints.

As we saw above, the prime supporters of the midtarsal complex are the tendons of the deep posterior compartment: tibialis posterior, flexor hallucis longus, and flexor digitorum longus. The flexor hallucis longus clearly helps lift the proximal part of the arch by supporting the sustentaculum tali. It then provides a tension wire along the entire medial aspect of the foot to the big toe, which also dorsiflexes as the foot progresses onto the toe rocker, further lengthening this line. The flexor hallucis longus is also crossed by the flexor digitorum longus, giving a suspension to the arch, especially during the toe rocker phase (see fig. 6.9).

The tibialis posterior is the last part of the supporting and balancing system of the foot from the lower leg. Its tendon attaches to all the middle metatarsals—second, third, and fourth—as well as to the bones comprising the bulk of the midtarsal joint complex: the navicular, all three cuneiforms, and the cuboid. So while the other tendons give distal (the two long toe flexors), medial (the tibialis anterior and fibularis longus) and lateral (the fibularis brevis) support, it is really the tibialis posterior that draws these central and more stable bones together (see fig. 6.9).

The tibialis posterior is challenged, however, by the positioning of its flat tendon under the malleolus, as this is an area of high stress at heel strike, which requires the absorption of the forceful rear foot eversion. This section of the tendon is hypovascular, and dysfunction can greatly affect the mechanics of the rest of the foot—and therefore the rest of the body!—and be slow and stubborn to correct.

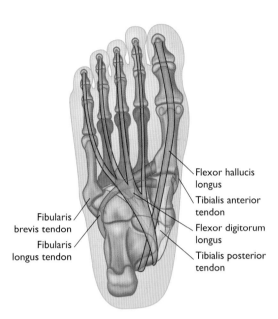

Flexor hallucis
longus

Tibialis anterior
tendon

Fibularis
brevis tendon

Flexor digitorum
longus

Fibularis
longus tendon

Tibialis posterior
tendon

Figure 6.9. The long tendons attaching to the plantar surface create a corrective system for the arches of the foot. The tibialis anterior and fibularis longus (red) form a sling. While they usually work in opposition to one another, they do cooperate to draw the base of the first metatarsal into the medial arch. The fibularis brevis does the same for the fifth metatarsal and the lateral arch. When both fibularii are tensioned by the dorsiflexion of the talar joint, the tibialis anterior will be shortened and will therefore require the support from the rest of the anterior Spiral Line (see chapter 5).

The two long toe flexors, hallucis and digitorum (*blue*), cross under the medial arch. As they are tensioned by the combined dorsiflexion of the ankle and toe rockers, they support and "approximate"—pull together—the distal ends, or at least they prevent them from spreading farther away.

The tibialis posterior (*yellow*) attaches to almost everything else, including the navicular, all three cuneiforms, and the cuboid, and it gives support to the three metatarsals not supported by the tibialis anterior or fibularis brevis. This strong corrector of pronation therefore crosses the midtarsal and tarsometatarsal joints of the second to fourth rays (*green*). These tarsometatarsal joints only allow dorsiflexion/plantarflexion; the first and fifth (*uncolored*) have more variation in their movements and are stabilized differently to allow this flexibility.

PUSH-OFF

Once the foot is brought back to the supinated position through the combination of inversion, lateral rotation, and dorsiflexion, the bones create a stable base to push from. In relaxed walking, however, we very rarely "push" during push-off; instead, we use most of the so-called plantarflexors in isometric contraction, as we saw with the gastrocnemius and soleus in the Superficial Back Line. So while they may be lengthening proximally in dorsiflexion, they are shortening distally to bring together the bones of the feet (the "econcentric" described in chapter 5). This form of contraction is necessary, as the proximal portion of all of these myofascial elements will be moving away from the distal insertions as the leg tilts forward to create the dorsiflexion (see fig. 6.10).

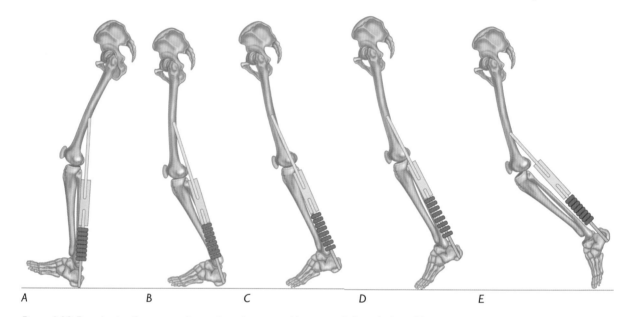

A   B   C   D   E

Figure 6.10. From heel strike, as we roll over the calcaneus and begin to roll through the ankle, we start to dorsiflex and lengthen the plantarflexors (A and B). This decelerates the lower leg, allowing the femur to move faster, with the swing of the other leg, and bring the knee into extension, as we roll onto the ball of the foot (C). Coming into toe dorsiflexion with the toe rocker (D) creates the final portion of the wind-up in the elastic tissue, which is released like a catapult mechanism in push-off (E).

Proprioceptors—the Internal Monitors

We actively "push off" when we need to walk faster or ascend a slope. At those times, the tension is constantly monitored and adjusted through the mechanoreceptors in the calf. In an ingenious experiment, Sawicki applied a mechanical boot with pneumatic "muscles" that assisted plantarflexion (Sawicki, Lewis, and Ferris 2009). It gave "free" energy to the subject's push-off phase, and the research team found that users quickly altered the amount of muscle force they used to adapt and compensate for the extra force coming from the boot. This allowed the subject to keep their walking kinematics relatively normal. "The user's nervous system reduced the triceps surae muscle activity in response to the mechanical assistance." Essentially, the demands of the job changed, and the proprioceptors adjusted the muscle effort accordingly.

What Sawicki, Lewis, and Ferris are saying is that our internal mechanoreceptors are able to constantly adjust in accordance with the mechanical forces involved in walking, keeping the muscle activity at a minimum to ensure maximum efficiency. Sawicki continued to explore the benefits of the architecture of muscles that allow this elastic mechanism and found that they tend to be pennate muscles with long tendons (see fig. 6.11). The pennation of muscles—in which the muscle fibers are attached to the tendons at an angle—allows a greater number of fibers to be included in the muscle unit. This allows a muscle to create more power, or, in this case, allows it to withstand more lengthening, so that the kinetic force goes into and loads the elastic tissues of the tendons (and the surrounding fascial elements).

Sawicki, Lewis, and Ferris appear to have focused their readings on the soleus muscle, as they were using surface EMG, but looking at the architecture of the other plantar flexors of the deep posterior compartment, we can clearly see that they all follow the same pattern of pennation with long tendons (see fig. 6.11, overleaf).

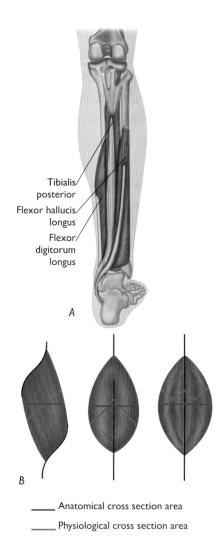

Tibialis
posterior

Flexor hallucis
longus

Flexor
digitorum
longus

A

B

_____ Anatomical cross section area

_____ Physiological cross section area

Figure 6.11. In the anatomy of the deep posterior calf muscles (A), we can see the angulation of the muscle fibers and their long, elastic tendons diving under the foot to join the phalanges and the tarsals. By using this arrangement, the muscles have a shorter range of motion than a fusiform muscle (a muscle with fibers that are parallel and run the full length of the unit). In cross section (B), we can see how we have to take a series of sections of a pennate muscle to count the actual number of fibers contained in a single unit, compared to the fusiform muscle, for which only one section is needed. The result of this is that the fusiform muscles have a longer range but produce less power than the shorter-range pennate muscles. In the case of our leg muscles, that power is used to encourage the kinetic energy to load the elastic fascial tissues. By holding isometric contractions, the muscle saves metabolic energy and stores kinetic energy for use in the catapult system.

HIP FLEXION

As mentioned above, a Z-shaped stretch is created by the combination of foot dorsiflexion and hip extension, and in exercise 6.1, one can feel the connection from the front of the pelvis to the medial arch of the foot. However, one can also feel the connection from the pelvis up through the upper body. In effect, the Deep Front Line is combining the production of hip flexion with plantarflexion, the same position in which we use the Superficial Front and Back Lines in chapter 3.

Exercise 6.2. Start by assuming the same position as in exercise 6.1—one leg back and internally rotated—and bring yourself to the "point of bind," where the medial arch of the back foot begins to lift.

Then bring your body further into a gentle thoracic extension, so your rib cage is up, but then exhale deeply to help relax the scalenes and the deep anterior neck tissue. Do you sense a change through the center of your body? Does it affect your back foot and its arch?

With this exercise you can also feel the effects of the different movements. More of one will restrict the other—for example, more thoracic extension can limit your ability to internally rotate your hip. Similarly, and perhaps more concerning, if there is not enough "loading" in one plane then another movement must be increased to compensate. A decrease in adduction or abduction may increase the need for extension, or for more work to be produced by the muscles involved.

The implication of this phenomenon is that too much movement in one plane may also limit the loading of tissues in another plane, while too little loading in one plane will increase the movement required in another—that is, insufficient loading, causing a lack of elastic recoil, will require more work from the muscles to aid the recovery. This is a central part of this book's thesis: the movement that occurs to lengthen the fascial tissue must be balanced. The most efficient movement is a "Goldilocks" event, with just the right amount of movement and load. This is true for all of the other areas we have looked at so far, and we will discuss in more detail in chapter 8.

The psoas is perhaps the muscle with the most conflicting descriptions—it is variously described as a strong hip flexor or not a hip flexor at all, an internal or external rotator, and an adductor or abductor of the hip. The truth is that it will do all of these things, depending on your starting position. As many have said before, when describing function, we must not limit ourselves to discussions based on anatomical position and the concentric/eccentric model of movement, the body is much more interesting than that. Unfortunately, it can be much more confusing also.

Gibbons summarizes much of the work that has been done on the function of the psoas in an attempt to gain some clarity (in Vleeming et al. 2007). Most investigations have shown the psoas to have little effect in movement of the lumbar spine, except perhaps in the production of lordosis, but it has quite consistently been found to create axial compression of the lumbar spine, meaning that when tensioned, the psoas helps stabilize the lower spinal segments. Gibbons also describes the fascial anatomy of the psoas as being continuous into the tissue of the transversus abdominis, internal oblique, and the pelvic floor, again emphasizing its potential role within this "core stability" complex.

Interestingly, however, Gibbons describes the psoas as being a unipennate muscle (i.e., it has one group of pennated, angled fibers) with shorter than expected muscle fibers, which he says questions "its efficiency as a hip flexor," as the fibers show no significant change of length. He posits that the iliacus is a more active flexor of the hip joint. As we saw above with the three tendons of the deep posterior compartment and the work of Sawicki, efficiency is increased by having a pennate structure. As the hip goes into extension, the muscle tissue of the psoas may be contracting to send the load into the elastic tissues, which will then recoil into flexion. At the same time, the mechanism will encourage a "force closure" of the lumbars. Compressing the lumbars as the hip goes into extension appears functionally sound, as it will increase the stability of the lower back as the body's center of gravity moves away from its base of support.

It therefore seems that the Z-stretch created in hip flexion/ankle dorsiflexion assists a force-closure form of stability at both ends of this line (see fig. 6.12). It helps to draw together the loose bones of the foot and stabilize the vulnerable lumbar spine. The use of pennate muscles allows the system the strength and efficiency to decelerate the forces of the body's momentum.

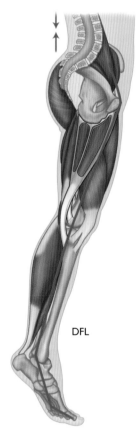

DFL

Figure 6.12. In this deliberately exaggerated view, you can see how the Z-stretch begins to draw together the less-stable bones of both the foot and the lumbar to create a force-closure effect and to produce a more stable platform for push-off.

DEEP FRONT LINE AT HEEL STRIKE AND A HEALTHY PELVIC FLOOR

The calcaneus prepares itself for heel strike by slightly inverting in the moments before the foot contacts the ground. Some of this is achieved by the tone within tibialis anterior, but that muscle's attachments on the base of the first metatarsal are quite far from the calcaneus, indicating there is another mechanism at work in the calcaneus's movement. This may involve the line of tension created from the adductor magnus to the deep posterior compartment. As the femur comes forward into flexion prior to the foot landing, adductor magnus is pre-tensioned, assisting the contractile efficiency to prevent further hip flexion (as we saw in the last chapter, with the biceps femoris). A mechanical force seems to be communicated across the knee and into the fascia of the deep posterior compartment that support medial arch (see fig. 6.13).

The fascia crossing the medial aspect of the knee may be able to communicate tension from both the flexor and extensor adductors to the foot, allowing them both to create some foot supination. At heel strike, however, that connection is very quickly lost, as the foot rapidly plantarflexes, the knee flexes, and the hip adducts. All of those movements will break the tension in the fascial continuity, despite the strong contraction of the adductor magnus.

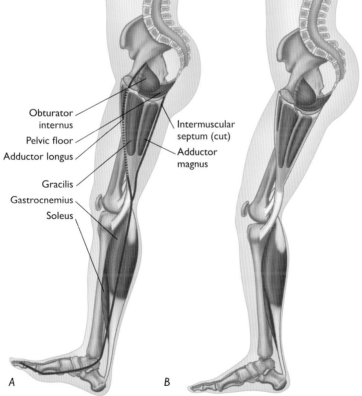

Obturator internus
Pelvic floor
Adductor longus
Gracilis
Gastrocnemius
Soleus

Intermuscular septum (cut)
Adductor magnus

A   B

Figure 6.13. A, Prior to heel strike, the posterior section of the DFL is tensioned via the combination of hip flexion, knee extension, and foot dorsiflexion, which allows the tissue of the adductor magnus to communicate to the myofascia supporting the medial arch. B, Heel strike causes rapid plantarflexion, knee flexion, and hip adduction (not shown here), all of which reduce the fascial communication across the joints.

After heel strike, the knee is driven across the front of the body, creating a knee valgus. The guy rope of the DFL, in crossing the inside of the knee, will also help push the knee back to neutral in the frontal plane, thereby correcting it from the valgus position (see fig. 6.14).

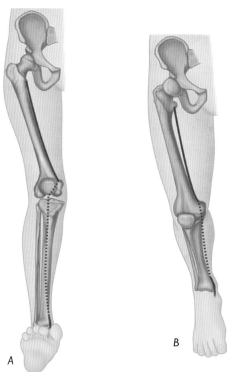

A

B

Figure 6.14. A, As the calcaneus tilts on heel strike, it forces the knee to move medially and thereby eccentrically loads this portion of the DFL. B, The tensioning of the myofascial line from the front of the pelvis to the medial longitudinal arch is created by hip extension and automatically corrects the fall of the arch.

The adductor magnus assists the hamstrings, the gluteus maximus, and the other hip extensors at heel strike. Its fascial continuity, however, is with the obturator internus on the other side of the ischiopubic ramus, and it may give us another method to decelerate the internal rotation of the femur. This could prove an interesting subject of future research: to look at the relation between these two muscles, which work together to stabilize the pelvis in flexion, but which oppose each another in rotation.

Following heel strike, the mechanical stimulus from the adductor magnus and obturator internus will carry tension to the pelvic floor and so to the psoas, with its continuity to the transversus abdominis. Thus, the adductor magnus may also be able to "switch on" the "core" system, especially in the pelvic floor. This is seen in the way the pelvic floor is initially tonified by the infant's many teetering experiments while learning to walk (see fig. 6.15).

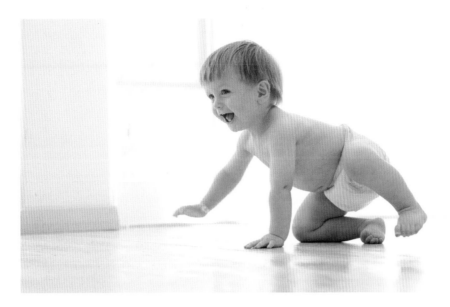

Figure 6.15. In the wobbling, unsteady process of the first attempts at walking, the toddler uses the adductors, which stimulates contractions and tone in the pelvic floor. This not only helps the child learn to stand and walk but also helps him or her establish urinary and fecal continence.

By stimulating a contraction within the walls of muscle that surround the abdominal cavity (the pelvic floor, the transversus abdominis, and the diaphragm), the body may take advantage of another hydraulic amplifier kind of mechanism (see fig. 6.16; see overleaf). Through the tension within the transversus abdominis, the body pre-tensions the epimysia—the sheath of tissue surrounding individual muscles—of the muscles that stabilize the lower back: the psoas, quadratus lumborum, erector spinae, and multifidi. These different layers of muscle may be receiving mechanical tension via the different layers of the thoracolumbar fascia: the psoas via the transversus abdominis and the anterior layer of the thoracolumbar fascia, due to the movements involving the Deep Front Line; the internal and external obliques via the Lateral and Spiral Line vectors that engage the middle layer of the thoracolumbar fascia.

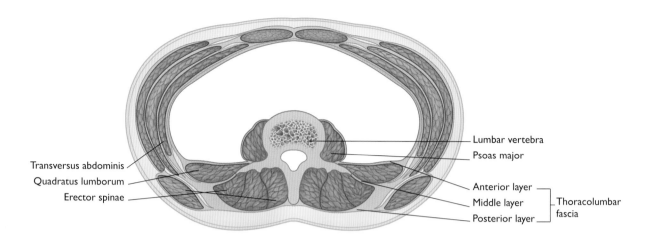

Transversus abdominis
Quadratus lumborum
Erector spinae

Lumbar vertebra
Psoas major

Anterior layer
Middle layer
Posterior layer

Thoracolumbar fascia

Figure 6.16. The contraction of adductor magnus at heel strike may stimulate the pelvic floor and transversus abdominis, tensioning the fascial layers surrounding the erector spinae, helping to stabilize the lower back and assisting the erectors. We will explore this further with the Back Functional Line in chapter 7.

FRONT AND BACK BALANCING

The posterior layer of the important thoracolumbar fascia is also the connection between the latissimus dorsi on one side of the body and the gluteus maximus on the opposite side, as discussed in chapter 5.

As the Spiral Line connects with the Back Functional Line via the switch at the greater trochanter, it forms the posterior section of the "Swingwalker" mechanism proposed by Zorn and Hodeck. In this model, Zorn and Hodeck suggest that an "inverted pendulum" model of gait requires the efficiency of elastic recoil on front and back (see fig. 6.17). As discussed earlier, the front of the body contributes significantly through the Superficial Front Line and the anterior portion of the Spiral Line. Both of these lines, however, take us from the femur and pelvis to the thoracic cage. The Deep Front Line follows a more profound path, bringing us to the inside of the ilium and the anterior lumbar spine, and connecting to the diaphragm via this internal route.

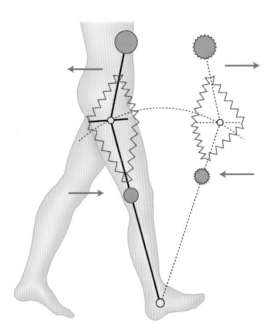

Figure 6.17. Rolfers and physicists Adjo Zorn and Kai Hodeck developed a computer-based model of walking. Expanding on previous works that looked at walking as a pendulum-type action, they realized the necessity of adding a second—and inverted—pendulum connected with two springs. If they correctly set the tension in the springs, the model was able to turn kinetic energy into elastic energy and thus produce a passive system of movement that required no engine (muscle) or other form of energy. Adapted from Hodeck and Zorn in Dalton et al 2011.

"We created a sagittal plane model in a computer program and endowed it with the precise anthropometric data.... We solved the movement equations with the help of some mathematical tools of applied mechanics and determined the spring parameters (length and stiffness) that make the design work properly" (Hodeck and Zorn in Dalton et al 2011).

The three-dimensional network of connective tissue, so richly endowed with mechanoreceptors, is the body's computer network. It is constantly receiving stimulation through movement, and—presumably through pattern recognition—it can adjust the muscle tone to make the correct response. Through repetition (how many times does a toddler fall down before he or she learns how to stand up, then cruise, then walk, then run?), it seems we learn the most efficient methods of moving—although many requisite elements are involved for that to occur, not just structural and functional aspects, but environmental and social aspects as well.

In efficient movement, Zorn and Hodeck suggest that the psoas in particular is the elastic element that works in opposition to the posterior sling of the Spiral Line and Back Functional Line. The psoas is given much credence for a lot of work, and, as discussed above, it complements many other fascial elements, especially that of the Superficial Front Line. The psoas is often greatly honored by bodyworkers for its central role within the body and for the fact that it acts as a conduit for the lumbar plexus. Could it be that its intimacy with the lumbar plexus helps in its "computations" in its part of the body's computer network?

ELASTIC EFFICIENCY MONITORING

Zorn and Hodeck's work gives us a valid (though computer-generated) model for how the body might be able to take advantage of reciprocal arrangements to encourage the efficiency of elastic recoil. Obviously, it is much more complex than the pelvis being able to bounce back and forth on a computer screen. However, the quote above can give us insight into the mechanical monitoring process that we saw earlier in Sawicki's mechanical plantarflexing boot, in which the plantarflexors adjusted the strength of their firing in concert with the work that was being produced by the boot. When plantarflexion was assisted, the muscles somehow "knew" to do less work.

We see this kind of internal and automatic adjustment occurring in other studies, such as studies that examined the force of heel strike with various amounts of cushioning. Essentially, the degree of protection offered to the foot changes the amount of force with which the foot hits the ground. This is what you can feel when you start using shoes with less cushioning after a few days of wearing more protective shoes: the first few steps are harder than normal. But the body quickly adapts, equalizing the forces with no conscious effort on your part.

A number of reasons have been put forward for this. I believe it allows us to optimize the amount of kinetic loading we receive into the body. If we land with too much force, the body cannot effectively absorb the shock; if we land too softly, the deceleration force required to absorb the shock is not strong enough to load the elastic tissue, forcing the body to use more energy to continue its movement—it is more energy inefficient to creep than to walk. And so, when working properly, the proprioceptors are looking for that "Goldilocks" level at which the kinetic energy is "just right" to load the elastic tissue and benefit from the elastic recoil to reduce active work.

Research by Snel shows that the forces at impact remain relatively stable regardless of the footwear used (see fig. 6.18) (cited in Gracovetsky, in Dalton 2011). While the study looked at running, it may also inform us about the change in heel strike impact following a sudden switch of footwear. Quite often when transitioning from cushioned to thinner soles, one can feel the shock of the heel strike for the first step or two, as the "computations" recalibrate the absorbing system.

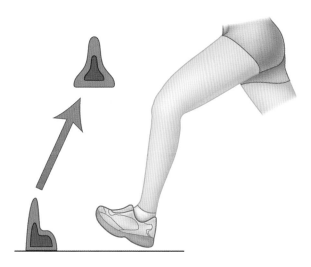

Figure 6.18. When investigating the heel strike pulse (P1), Snel showed that using a variation of footwear with different paddings (as well as being barefoot) made very little difference to the heel strike pulse. It was proposed that the body adjusts its movement to maintain a relatively consistent loading through the tissue.

ESSENTIAL EVENTS

As the previous chapter has already covered each of the three planes of motion—sagittal with the SFL and SBL, frontal with the LTL, and transverse with the SPL—most of the events are now accounted for. There are a few specific to the DFL, which are outlined below, but the important point for the Deep Front Line is that all of the superficial lines are able to load simultaneously.

Our aim should be to ensure an even load through each of the lines so that no one line has to produce more work or absorb more stress than any other. The superficial lines must be long enough to let the momentum of movement load the deeper tissue, they also must be strong enough to absorb their fair share of the forces involved. Dysfunction will result from imbalances in the "stiffness absorbing system" of the myofascia, caused by overuse or underuse. To correct dysfunction, one must find ways of using strengthening and stretching exercises that target the appropriate tissue, while also recognizing the role of the proprioceptors—not all dysfunction is caused by tissue limitations, it can be caused by motor patterning.

Gently encouraging clients into the essential events can tell you whether movement restrictions are proprioceptive or actual tissue limitations. We often learn bad habits, failing to use the full length of our myofascia through movement patterns caused by previous injuries or simply by wanting to mimic the movement of someone close to us. These bad habits can train our mechanoreceptors to use patterns that are not ideal for fascial efficiency, requiring more work and/or creating imbalance at the transition points of heel strike and push-off. Figures for the number of repetitions required before a movement becomes a habit vary, but hover around three hundred. The figure for removing or changing that habit is around three thousand, making it ten times more difficult to unlearn a pattern than to learn it.

Z Stretch and Hip Position

As you felt in the two exercises above (6.1 and 6.2), the engagement of the anterior DFL plays an important role at the point of push-off. Unlike the SBL and SFL, the DFL will be involved in both plantarflexion and hip flexion, tasks ascribed to the SBL and SFL, respectively.

For a fully effective engagement of the psoas tendon, the psoas needs to be properly elongated, a position achieved by the extended hip being abducted and internally rotated relative to the pelvis. Not only is the tendon's distal attachment being lengthened, but the proximal attachment on the diaphragm will also be side flexing to the opposite side (see fig. 6.19).

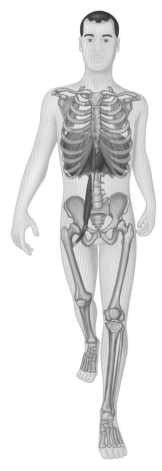

Figure 6.19. This slightly exaggerated outline shows how the hip and lumbar movements conspire to allow for full elastic loading of the psoas tendon. As discussed above, not only will this assist with push-off, but it may also contribute to lumbar stability, important in those moments of greatest challenge, at the extreme ends of normal range. The psoas manages to perform two tasks in one movement—the countermovement of the lower limb and stabilization of the lower back.

Heel Whip

A short and quick medial "whip" of the heel at push-off is a common indicator of restriction in the psoas. The internal rotation at the hip drives a strong force into the flexor complex—perhaps beyond its easy range—overwinding the tissue in the transverse plane. This energy is suddenly released at push-off. It makes itself visible by the small but significant external rotation of the limb, which, when viewed from the back, is seen as a fast medial movement of the calcaneus. This "whip" may create callouses on the forefoot and rotational wear patterns on the soles of any footwear.

In recalcitrant cases of this problem, it is also worthwhile to check the fibularii, which—being synergistic with the psoas in their effect on the foot—can also produce a similar force.

Postural Considerations

Maintaining an upright stance influences DFL in a positive way. The connections from the jaw and throat into the thoracic cavity and on to the diaphragm seem able to create a proximal tensioning of the hip flexors. The sprinter Michael Johnson ran with his back extended and his chin tucked in, apparently taking advantage—to great effect—of the extra recoil available from the anterior lines (see fig. 6.20).

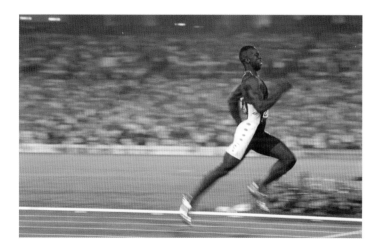

Figure 6.20. Michael Johnson's running style for the 200 and 400 meters was revolutionary at the time. His upright stance, combined with shorter strides, was perhaps maximizing the elastic recoil through the Deep Front Line to speed hip flexion. Photograph courtesy of Getty Images.

An anterior head position, a collapsed rib cage, and any rotations and tilts in the spine may all negatively influence the flow of tensions in the DFL, which will contribute to imbalances in all of the other lines. The task is to learn to identify these postural problems and to make the appropriate changes through directed interventions—exercise, stretching, and soft-tissue manipulation, as necessary.

7 Arm and Functional Lines

If we select any object from the whole extent of animated nature, and contemplate it fully and in all its bearings, we shall certainly come to this conclusion: that there is design in the mechanical construction, benevolence in the endowments of the living properties, and that good on the whole is the result.
—Charles Bell, *1837, The Hand, Its Mechanisms and Vital Endowments,*
as Evincing Design

Whether we see the body as evolved or designed (as Charles Bell did), I think we would all agree on the wonderful job done on the upper girdle. The dexterity of the hand and the range of motion of the shoulder are both excellent schemes, allowing so many of our human abilities.

A contemporary of Bell's, Richard Lovejoy, is credited with being the first to notice that the schema for upper and lower limbs are virtually identical. And, as any visitor to the Natural History Museum in London, which Lovejoy founded, will see, this is not exclusive to humans: just about every other animal that has limbs follows the similar pattern: scapula/pelvis, humerus/femur, ulna and radius/tibia and fibula. There is much more variation in the carpals, tarsals, and phalanges, depending on the digitation strategy (hoofed, webbed, fingered, and so forth), but the overall building blocks are the same (see fig 7.1, overleaf).

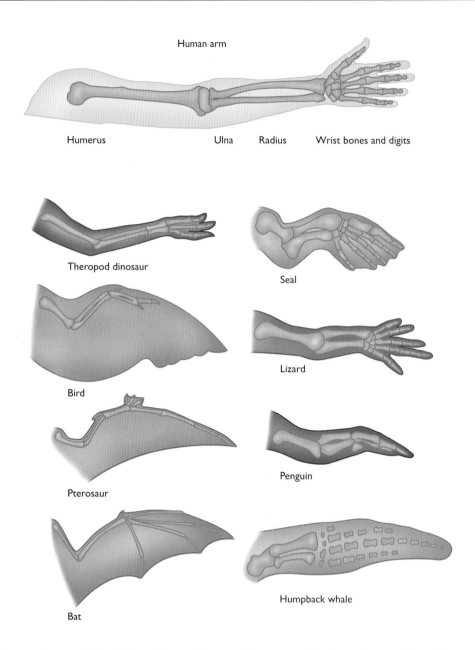

Figure 7.1. The general pattern of upper-limb architecture follows a similar pattern of one bone, then two, followed by a series of smaller bones in various arrangements.

Paleontologist Neil Shubin recently published his work on the discovery of Tiktaalik, a fossil found in 2004 on Ellesmere Island, Canada, and dated to 375 million years ago (see fig. 7.2). Tiktaalik is hugely significant, as it is a transition fossil, the remains of an amphibian that had the beginnings of jointed arms and a cervical spine. Before Tiktaalik was discovered, Shubin, after a study of other specimens, had predicted that these features should be found in fossils from approximately 375 MYA, and, after hunting down geological areas that would have encountered the correct weather patterns at that period, he found Tiktaalik—the missing link between earlier fossils that had developed an upper arm and upper thigh (380 MYA) and those with wrist and ankle bones (365 MYA).

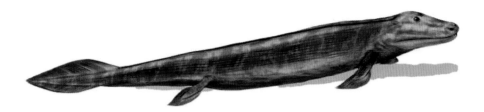

Figure 7.2. The famous fossil Tiktaalik (the name is Inuit for freshwater fish), which shows a flat head (a change from the conical fish head), a cervical spine, and a distinct upper limb. This fossil is widely hailed as illustrating the successful transition from sea to land.

While not claiming Tiktaalik to be our direct ancestor, just a distant cousin, Shubin does describe how humans came to develop these similar features via our Hox genes, which determine our basic shape and architecture. Slight variations in Hox genes lead to the changes we see in body shape, such as those discovered by Edward Lewis in his manipulation of the genes of the fruit fly *(Drosophila melanogaster)*, which produced mutations and rearrangements in body segments. This section of DNA shows very little variation across species throughout the animal kingdom and therefore seems to contain the essential coding for consistent body shape—which explains the general homology noticed by Lovejoy.

It is interesting that whatever mutation led to the development of the upper limb seems to have happened at around the same time as the separation of the head from the thorax via the cervical spine. Before 375 MYA, there was no such thing as a neck, which is quite an unstable arrangement, especially if plonking 8 percent of your body weight on top of it. This linked evolution must therefore be significant, and it should be taken into account when looking at the functional anatomy of the region.

The arm lines appear to give us the ability to use the weight of the upper girdles to assist the newly unstable head on top of its perch, while the functional lines provide a connection between the upper and lower limbs. Both of these arrangements, as might be expected from their recent development, are superficial to the older "core" that we saw with the Deep Front and Lateral Lines.

ARM LINES

There has been much debate on the role of the arms during gait. Everyone seems to accept that there is a contralateral swing with the lower limb, but there is little agreement on the reasons for this. Some believe the swing to be actively driven, others argue that it is a passive reaction to the rotation created by the legs.

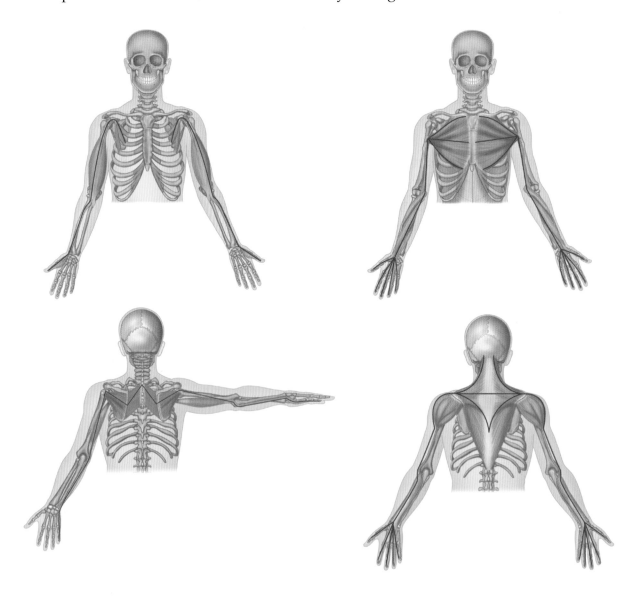

Figure 7.3. The upper girdles show four distinct myofascial continuities. However, the arm portions serve us less in walking; they come into their own during many other functional activities.

In Anatomy Train terms, the arm lines are not overly involved in walking, because the arms are never placed into a position to engage or stretch the full lines. This is especially true of the Deep Front Arm Line and Deep Back Arm Line (DFAL and DBAL), which have to "turn" at the glenohumeral joint (from the pectoralis minor and the rotator cuff muscles respectively) to descend along the arm with the biceps (DFAL) and triceps (DBAL). The Deep Back Arm Lines become more engaged with the other lines of the body when the arms are brought up into abduction and/or flexion or extension beyond 90 degrees, at which point the alignment of the fascicles become parallel (see fig. 7.4).

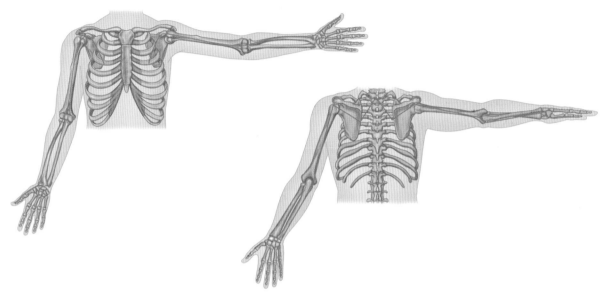

Figure 7.4. With the arm elevated in the frontal and/or sagittal plane, the tissues of the deep arm lines can cooperate to give extra stability and force distribution for activities such as throwing, catching, swinging, and pulling.

The two superficial arm lines appear to be more involved in walking, but seem to work in quite different ways. The Superficial Front Arm Line (SFAL) is intertwined with the Front Functional Line (FFL)—both will be addressed below. The Superficial Back Arm Line (SBAL) appears to play a role, as part of the upper girdle, in stability of the head.

Arm Swing and the Superficial Back Arm Line

A recent study by Pontzer, Holloway, Raichlen, and Lieberman found, as we would expect, that the deltoid is activated during arm swing (2009). What we may not have expected is that each portion of the deltoid contracts in response to the swing—not to create it. Both the anterior and posterior deltoid are working during the eccentric phase rather than contracting concentrically to initiate the arm movement. The countermovement is once again acting as the stimulus to the muscle fiber, which contracts to decelerate the motion and tension the fascial tissue. Pontzer went on to show that much of the movement of the upper limb is a response created by the stride of the legs and that the upper limb is predominately acting as a damper of the rotational forces created through the body.

While the study investigated the kinematics of walking (the shape and relationship of the bones) and took EMG readings, it only did so for the deltoid muscle, part of the Superficial Back Arm Line. Measurements were taken with subjects with different levels of arm swing (no swing, normal swing, and weighted swing) both when they were running and walking. The study showed that arm swing reduced the amount of movement of the head, especially when extra weight was added to the arms. Having no arm swing increased upper body movement by approximately 50 percent, showing that the upper girdle greatly helps to stabilize the head.

The study by Pontzer supports the theories of Harvard paleoanthropologist Daniel Lieberman, who suggests that the low, wide shoulders of *Homo sapiens,* coupled with the strong ligamentum nuchae, assist in reducing the ground reaction forces coming to the head. The ligamentum nuchae (which is formed from the interspinous ligaments and the blending of the trapezius muscles) plays a particularly important role.

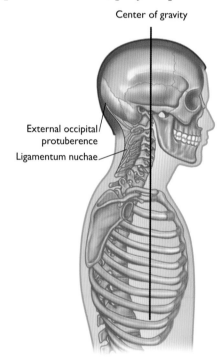

Center of gravity

External occipital
protuberence

Ligamentum nuchae

Figure 7.5. The ligamentum nuchae is also significant for support of the head for humans. The skulls of many of our hominid antecessors do not show the tuberosity of the external occipital protuberance. Lieberman hypothesizes that the change in our shoulder girdles, which are wider and lower than those of other hominids, helped develop the ligament, which assists with elastic stability of the head.

When we look at the order of the parts of the Superficial Back Arm Line we can see that the deltoid is a continuation of the trapezius; in fact, all of its proximal attachments match those of the distal trapezius. Though any textbook will list them on opposite sides of the clavicle and scapula, Myers has shown the tissue to be continuous across those bones.

This gives the contraction of the deltoid during arm swing a direct connection to the head and the neck ligament, allowing the head to utilize the energy of the moving arm for its stabilization. As Pontzer showed, take away arm swing, and the pitch and yaw of the head increases. Lieberman also states that the anterior (cleidocranial) portion of the trapezius contracts just prior to heel strike, which links the mass of the arm to the back of the head and helps prevent the head from pitching forward at impact (2011). As he points out, we need this mechanism, because the head's center of gravity is in front of the atlanto-occipital joint; extra support behind the axis helps maintain the head's anterior gaze (see fig. 7.5).

Chapter 5 showed how the Spiral Line connects the pelvis to the head via the shoulder girdle. The "newer" shoulder musculature of the upper limb, on quite a separate layer to that of the "fish" body, allows the contralateral rotation between the upper and lower limbs and assists with head stability in the transverse plane. Because the rhomboids and the splenii muscles attach through the ligamentum nuchae, they may also tension it, giving further assistance to the trapezius in preventing the forward pitch of the head in the sagittal plane.

FUNCTIONAL LINES

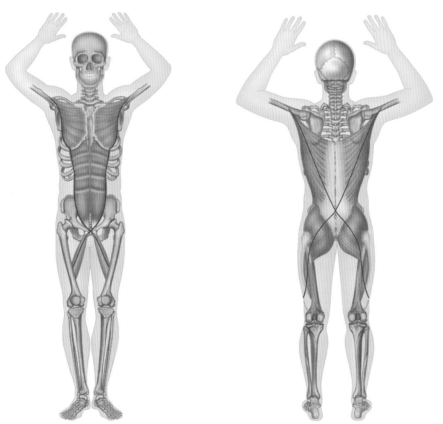

Figure 7.6. The Front Functional Line (FFL) overlaps with the Superficial Front Line and the Deep Front Line to use the humerus (along with the opposite femur) at push-off. The Back Functional Line (BFL) falls into the vector of force associated with the Spiral Line at heel strike (see chapter 5).

Front Functional Line

At the moment of push-off, with a contralateral arm swing, the opposite humerus should be at its furthest point from the leg that's pushing off. The pectoralis major will be contracting slightly to decelerate the arm's backswing, and this may allow the arm to create more tension through the Front Functional Line to load the elastic tissue (see fig. 7.7).

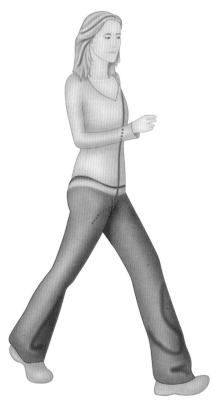

Figure 7.7. At push-off, the Front Functional Line will be engaged on one side via thoracic extension, hip abduction, and the backswing of the opposite humerus. This position tensions the costal fibers of the pectoralis major, leading into the rectus abdominis and finally into the adductor longus to the femur, which can then, along with the other lines, return the body toward the reverse position.

Just as the position of the head can affect recoil in the Superficial Front Line, as discussed in chapter 3, a similar (though smaller) effect can be felt when the arms either swing out of synch or not at all.

In Pontzer's research, the presence or absence of arm swing made no difference to the metabolic cost of walking. This does not necessarily negate the use of recoil and its communication through the tissue from the upper body to the lower. It is likely that the studies done so far have not been sophisticated enough to simultaneously measure elastic loading and other compensatory strategies the body may employ when one mechanism is taken away.

For example, they state, "running may lead to greater stabilizing muscle activity, and therefore a stronger linkage (i.e., a stiffer 'spring') between the pelvis, shoulder, and arm. Stiffer 'springs' may also be necessitated by the greater stride frequencies used in running, since stiffer springs would increase the natural frequencies for the body segments involved." In other words, the body adapts to the forces acting through it, adjusting the stiffness (when possible) to optimize efficiency. Once again, the myofascia is proving to be self-monitoring, making unconscious calibrations of the soft tissue and using the contractile properties of the muscles as a "stiffness adjusting system."

It is obvious that almost all adults can walk with or without arm swing, and while the evidence of its contribution to walking (as opposed to its reaction to the movement) has yet to be found, most walkers have felt the benefits and effects. Our conclusion must be that "more research is necessary" if we want to fully comprehend the downward chain of events from the shoulders.

Back Functional Line

In chapter 5 we saw how the Back Functional Line is recruited at heel strike to help the Spiral Line decelerate pronation: it creates a contralateral sling from one humerus to the opposite femur. This relationship has been well investigated by Vleeming and by Zorn. It is worthwhile to look now at how the Back Functional Line interacts with the deeper musculature of the back.

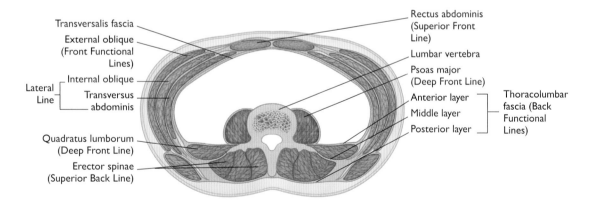

Figure 7.8. At heel strike, the Back Functional Line will be tensioned across the low back by hip flexion and opposite arm swing. This pre-tension will assist the deceleration of pronation but will also create a pressure into the erectors. The erectors (especially on the side of the extended leg) will be contracting in their vertical alignment quite strongly and so expanding their volume outward. Both quadrati lumborum will be contracting, dealing with the side flexions and rotations of the transverse processes on both sides. The internal and external obliques and the transversus abdominis will be tensioned by the trunk extension, side flexion, and rotation, and will therefore tension all of the anterior and middle layers of the thoracolumbar fascia. The lower back is a complex arrangement of myofascia contracting and gliding in different directions, and the contraction of each muscle assists the contraction of its neighbors through the hydraulic amplifier effect and parallel pre-tensioning of the tissue.

By contracting and by being pre-tensed in many different directions at heel strike, the lumbar complex can be viewed as an interdependent system (see fig. 7.8). The expansion of one muscle tenses the fascia of another, and the lengthening of the fascia created by the position at heel strike will add more power to the contraction. The distribution of fascial tension was investigated by Franklyn-Miller (2009). By performing a straight leg raise on five cadavers with devices that measured strain at appropriate points, they were able to record the amount of strain created through the leg and lower back (see fig. 7.9).

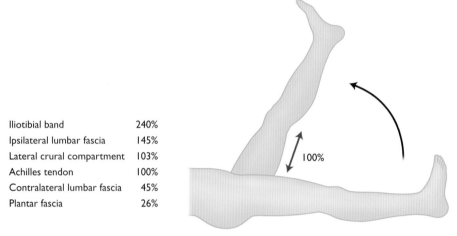

Iliotibial band	240%
Ipsilateral lumbar fascia	145%
Lateral crural compartment	103%
Achilles tendon	100%
Contralateral lumbar fascia	45%
Plantar fascia	26%

Figure 7.9. Using strain receptors placed on the listed sections, Franklyn-Miller demonstrated the strain distribution into the myofascial tissue when performing a straight leg raise. The research was performed on cadavers, showing the tensioning of the tissue was mechanical and not the result of muscular contraction. The results show the ability of hip flexion to create tension through the Superficial Back, Spiral, Lateral, and Back Functional Lines, and they also show the wider distribution of that tension—beyond the so-called muscle attachments of the hip extensors.

The tissue strain occurs at various depths within the body, and each layer needs to be able to move or glide and to facilitate movement beyond the section shown in figure 7.8. Thankfully, each of the septa between the muscles is "lubricated" by the areolar (loose connective) tissue. This tissue is a hydrated and malleable extension of the fascial system, and it allows the layers to glide on one another while maintaining their connection.

Ipsilateral Functional Line

In the second edition of "Anatomy Trains," Myers added the Ipsilateral Functional Line (IFL), which goes from the lateral aspect of the latissimus dorsi to the external obliques and onto the sartorius. While it is said to be involved in the crawl stroke in swimming, this line may have a more everyday use in its contribution to leg swing after push-off.

If we look at the lateral tissue at push-off, we see that the hip and knee are extended and the hip internally rotated, an ideal loading position for the sartorius (see fig. 7.10). The trunk will be relatively side flexed to the opposite side with the arm forward, also ideal for loading the latissimus dorsi and the lateral external obliques.

The resultant elastic loading will be increased by the firing of the external obliques to control the drop of the right ilium, and, once end of range is met, the whole line will then encourage the femur to laterally rotate, the knee and hip to flex (all actions of the sartorius), the right ilium to lift and rotate to the left (external obliques) and finally the shoulder girdle to rotate to the left and the humerus to extend (latissimus dorsi).

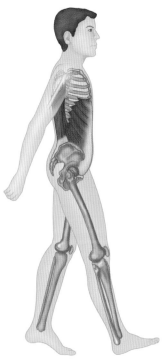

Figure 7.10. The lateral fibers of the latissimus dorsi will be tensioned by both the arm swing into flexion and the rotation of the shoulder girdle to the opposite side. The almost vertical fibers of the external oblique will be tensioned by the ilium dropping and rotating in the opposite direction from the shoulder girdle.

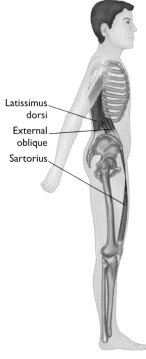

Latissimus dorsi

External oblique

Sartorius

Figure 7.11. Clearly seen in this dissection, the costal attachments of the latissimus dorsi carry into the lateral external obliques, which bring us to the anterior superior iliac spine and the sartorius.

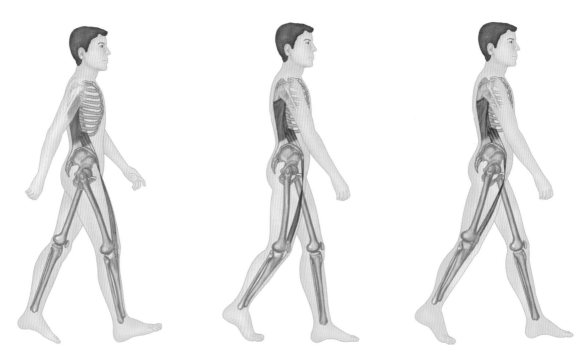

Figure 7.12. With the right Ipsilateral Functional Line naturally shortened due to the hip being flexed, the knee extended, and the shoulder girdle more vertically aligned with the continuity of the latissimus dorsi and external obliques, the leg is more able to "fall" into its loading pattern. With the progression into hip extension during swing phase and the shoulder girdle recoiling in the opposite direction, we see the gradual tensioning of this line, which can assist with the uncoiling of the leg rotation and can lead to the knee flexion required during the next swing phase.

SUMMARY

1. Arm swing dissipates the energy of the rotational forces caused by bipedal gait.

2. The Arm Lines are less involved with walking, as they are not engaged throughout their full line.

3. The trapezius and deltoid of the Superficial Front Arm Line help to stabilize the head in the sagittal plane through the ligamentum nuchae.

4. The Front Functional Line overlaps with the Superficial Front and Deep Front Lines to use the humerus position to assist the hip flexion at push-off.

5. The Back Functional Line blends into the Spiral Line (as discussed in chapter 6) at heel strike, using the greater trochanter as a "switch."

6. The myofascial complex of the lower back can be seen as an interdependent system using fascial tension and muscle contraction to assist the efficiency of the surrounding muscles.

7. All of this system requires the mobility between the layers provided by the loose connective tissue.

ESSENTIAL EVENTS

Arm Swing

While the debate on arm swing may be ongoing, we can still use its amplitude and rhythm as an indicator of what may be going on in other regions. Too much swing can be indicative of not enough rotational ability within the trunk, which would make the arms receive more than their normal share. If there is too much swing, check the thoracic rotation ability. If this appears normal, the length of the stride may be too long. It may also be worth investigating other factors: are the arms passive or are they being "driven" to create more swing? If the latter appears to be the case, investigating the historical and/or psychological motivation behind the excessive arm swing may uncover useful insights.

Front Functional Line

If the arm swing is normal and all of the "essential events" are in place, the Front Functional Line should be able to do its job. The main events in this line would be hip extension and adduction, thoracic extension, with relative rotation between the pelvis and thorax and opposite arm extension.

Back Functional Line

This is almost the exact opposite of the Front Functional Line. Here we need hip flexion, posterior tilt of the ilium on the same side, and rotation between the pelvis and the opposite shoulder girdle, coupled with arm flexion.

Ipsilateral Functional Line

For this lateral tissue to engage, the hip and knee must be extended and internally rotated; the pelvis must be tilted to the same side, and the arm flexed.

8 Spring Walker: Pull Me, Push You

Did man possess the natural armour of the brutes, he would no longer work as an artificer, nor protect himself with a breast-plate, nor fashion a sword or spear, nor invent a bridle to mount the horse and hunt the lion. Neither could he follow the arts of peace, construct the pipe and the lyre, erect houses, place altars, inscribe laws, and through letters and the ingenuity of the hand hold communion with the wisdom of antiquity, at one time converse with Plato, at another with Aristotle, or Hippocrates.
—Galen

The effectiveness of our bipedal gait has been honed and matured by evolution over the last 4 million years. Walking on two legs was something of a compromise of mobility over stability, because, by standing upright, we put our low backs and sacroiliac joints at some peril, but the advantages outweighed these occasional sacrifices.

Coming onto two legs may have decreased our exposure to the sun, and it certainly freed our arms for the control of tools and, eventually, fire. It is metabolically cheaper, allowing us to scavenge further from our home base. The development of running and, therefore, persistence hunting may have coincided with the capacity for abstract thought—being able to visualize and predict the movement of the hunted animal. Cooking the meat over the fire and sharing thoughts about the hunt (and then stories about it)—along with the cooperation necessary for the hunt itself—may have helped expand our early language.

All of these factors added to our adaptability, thereby to making calories more available to us. We have had larger, stronger, and bigger-brained cousins as ancestors, but we are the ones still around. As the dinosaurs learned—at their cost—bigger is not necessarily better. Our brawnier cousins, the Neanderthals, died out as well. They were sturdier and stronger than *Homo sapiens*, but probably required more calories to survive and presumably were not as agile.

Soft tissues are rarely, if ever, preserved in the fossil record, so we have no way of knowing exactly the difference between our elastic tissue and theirs. But judging from the solidity of Neanderthal bones and those bones' growth patterns and the insertion points, it seems clear that our lighter frame benefits from our fascial system. Our upright stance allows us to load the fascial system through gravity and through forward, backward, lateral, and rotational movement. We benefit from our unstable vertical alignment by letting it challenge and stretch the elastic tissues throughout the body, loading them with energy that we then use for movement, most commonly for walking.

Our survival, however, has been dependent on so much more. With just the minimum tools in terms of muscle power and strength, we have maximized our diversity. As I write, London is about to launch the 2012 Olympic Games, and while *Homo sapiens* will never outrun a cheetah, lift more weight than a rhino, or swim faster than a dolphin, it is a fact that we can perform all of these activities. Disney may have created a form of animal games in the 1973 film *Robin Hood*, the fact remains that that could only be done in animation. No other animal has mastered such a wide range of movement in such a variety of different environments.

Our versatility is unmatched, and we do most motions (once practiced!) with grace, with an ease that is the hallmark of fascial efficiency. As Fukashiro states, "Most dynamic movements in sports activities involve a countermovement, where an agonist muscle contracts after being stretched in an eccentric phase, which is usually defined as a stretch shortening cycle" (2006). Essentially, by going in the direction opposite from the one we want to travel in, we are using the efficient dynamics of stretch shortening cycle, which is "the natural way of muscle function in normal locomotion … nature's way to combine the available resources … in such a way that both peak performance and movement economy are considered in the most appropriate way in each particular movement situation" (Komi 2011).

When we match joint alignment with the pull of gravity and the ground reaction force—coupled with the momentum involved in any movement—we can see how the dynamics are channeled into the elastic tissues. By exploiting the instability of our vertical alignment and smooth joints, we easily gain countermovement. The proprioceptors embedded within our wonderful three-dimensional web of fascial tissue activate the necessary muscles to decelerate the action that stretches the elastic fascial tissue, which can assist the recovery movement with metabolically "free" energy.

When we look at Muybridge's horse progressing from a trot to a gallop, we see increases in flexion and extension, the greater movement putting more load into the tissues to support and produce the stronger forces required. The quadruped is more clearly a full-body walker; the quote that began this book shows that we have yet to appreciate the full involvement of our anatomy in locomotion, since half of it is sadly labeled the "passenger" (Perry and Burnfield 2010).

I think it is an interesting exercise to take the two transition points—heel strike and push-off—and reverse-engineer them by simply looking at where the forces are traveling. At push-off, we have progressed our pelvis forward from the back foot to create a line of tension along the entire front of the body:

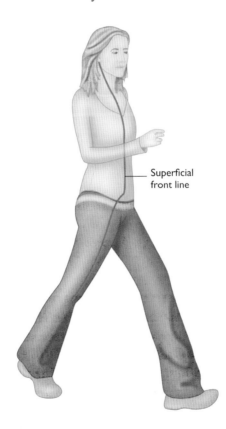

Superficial front line

Figure 8.1. The extended position at push-off stretches most of the anterior tissues of the body, we just happen to call it the Superficial Front Line. So by going into extension, we have put kinetic energy into many of the flexors to be released at push-off.

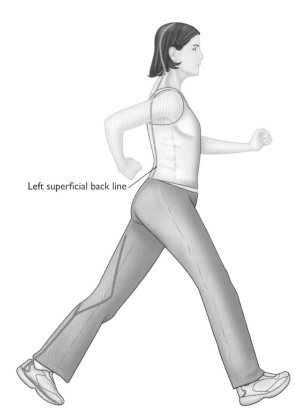

Left superficial back line

Figure 8.2. While the Superficial Front Line is shorter in the lower portion at the front of the ankle, the dorsiflexion and knee extension have stretched the lower portion of the Superficial Back Line.

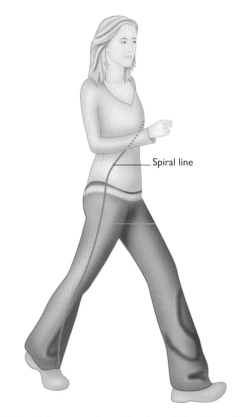

Spiral line

Figure 8.3. The counterrotation of the shoulder girdle creates the tension through the oblique Spiral Line, which, through the tensor fascia lata and tibialis anterior, will assist hip flexion and foot supination. The same position will follow the Front Functional Line for extra support to the extended femur.

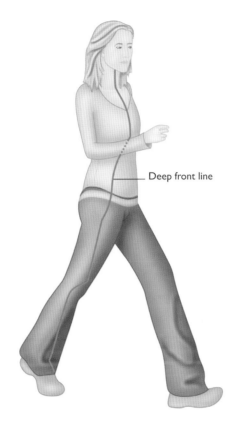

Deep front line

Figure 8.4. The combination of dorsiflexion, knee extension, hip extension, abduction, and internal rotation is the ideal position to lengthen the Deep Front Line, which will assist with almost all the required events at push-off.

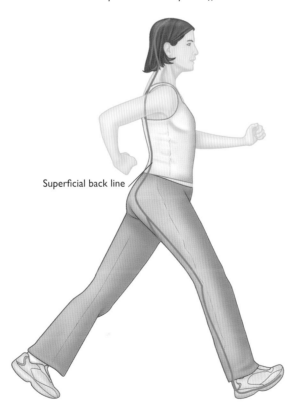

Superficial back line

Figure 8.5. At heel strike, the flexed hip position will require support from all of the hip extensors. They will be in a pre-tensioned position due to the flexion, the Superficial Back Line will be further lengthened by the ankle dorsiflexion.

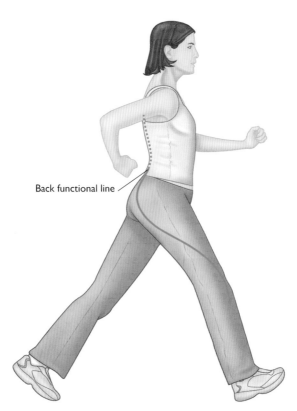

Back functional line

Figure 8.6. The Spiral Line overlaps with the Superficial Back Line in its use of the biceps femoris, but at heel strike, we can follow the rotational forces caused by the tilt of the calcaneus to bring us to the superior portion of the gluteus maximus from the tibialis anterior and the iliotibial band. From there we carry into the latissimus dorsi to create a form of sling (as used by Zorn and Vleeming). This superficial sling addresses the rotational aspects of the pronation pattern, while the deeper posterior portion of the Spiral Line helps balance the sacroiliac joint through the connection to the sacrotuberous ligament and the long dorsal sacroiliac ligament on the opposite side.

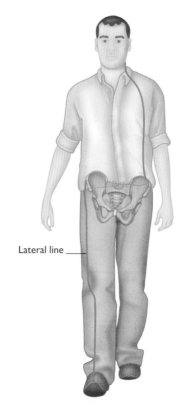

Lateral line

Figure 8.7. With the center of gravity at the midline of the body offset from the point of support, the hip is encouraged into adduction on the side of heel strike, which loads the lower Lateral Line on that side. Meanwhile, the upper Lateral Line is opened on the opposite flank.

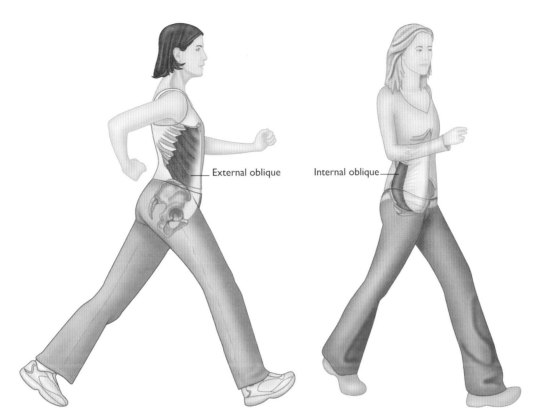

Figure 8.8. With the pelvis moving farther and faster than the rib cage, the Xs of the Lateral Line will be stretched in opposite directions on each side. These "ipsilateral" obliques therefore carry the rotation created by bipedal gait into the intercostals—this is dampened by the counterrotation of the arms and the "contralateral" obliques of the Spiral Line/Front Functional Line (see fig. 8.3).

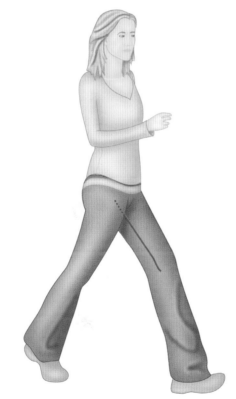

Figure 8.9. As the leg swings through into hip flexion, the adductor magnus on the swing leg will be lengthened, in order to pre-tension it prior to heel strike, when it will work to resist further flexion. During the swing phase, it may help to tension the deep posterior compartment fascia to supinate the foot prior to heel strike.

If we look back to the work of Huijing, mentioned in chapter 1, in which he examined the transfer of force from one tendon into the surrounding tissue, we can now really appreciate the complexity and beauty of the myofascial arrangements. Working as a separator, connector, force concentration and dispersal system, the myofascial system not only communicates mechanical information directly through its fibers but also senses and adjusts the sectional stiffness according to the forces acting at any one time.

FOOTWEAR

Nature, Mr. Allnut, is what we are put in this world to rise above.
—Rose Sayer (played by Katharine Hepburn) in *The African Queen*

One of the most obvious ways we try to rise above nature is through adornment, and, when not passing our time inventing new methods of maiming and killing each other, humanity has often diverted its attention to novel ways of mutilating the body we inherited. From foot binding to winklepickers, stilettos to platform boots, each generation and each culture has managed to find a way to interfere with the natural dynamics of our feet. When left to their own devices, our feet serve us quite well, and they really need little more than some protective covering to save us from the vagaries of litter and sharp (or sometimes squidgy) objects.

Hopefully by this stage of the book, enough evidence of the interaction between anatomy, function, and evolution has been presented to convince you of their interrelationship.

So, with apologies to Miss Sayer, we would be better served by not trying to rise above our nature, at least in the foot department. A thick sole will dampen our proprioceptive feedback (Saxby 2011). An elevated heel will force more of the body weight onto the metatarsal heads, stressing them, and it will shorten the Achilles tendon, distorting the posture and interfering with the communication through the lines. An elevation of two inches will give the body an incline of 20 degrees, leading to a 23 percent increase in the load on the front of the knees. A three-inch heel puts 76 percent of the body weight on the metatarsal heads, which are not designed for that kind of constant stress (see fig. 8.10).

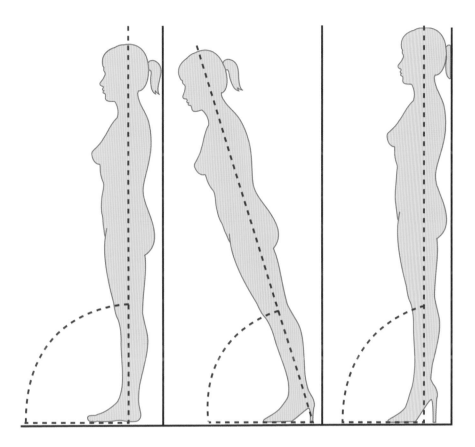

Figure 8.10. A, The incline of the heel has to be compensated for somewhere in the body: at the knee, the hips, the lumbar spine, or the thoracic spine, depending on one's tendency. This places undue stress on any or all of those areas, increasing the likelihood of pain and dysfunction. B, As the heel increases in height, an ever-greater percentage of body weight is brought to the ball of the foot, decreasing efficiency and increasing stress on the bones. Adapted from Dalton 2011.

Cramped toe boxes lead to misalignment of the first and fifth toes (predominately, though in many cases the others can be affected as well), which leads to varied angles at push-off (see fig. 8.11, see overleaf). This can be further exacerbated by the longitudinal axis of the shoe, which is often curved, especially in athletic shoes.

If you want to forget all your other troubles, wear too tight shoes.
—*The Houghton Line*, **November 1965**

For a normal foot, the ideal shoe would be flat (see fig. 8.11*B*). Wearing a minimal sole allows clear proprioception, but it should be thick enough and strong enough to offer protection. A wider toe box gives the toes room to spread on contact with the ground, which is mechanically useful. As the metatarsals spread, the interossei will be stretched, signaling a reflex contraction of the quadriceps (Michaud 2011). A simple arrangement of the shoe, one in which the alignment of the foot is unaltered, is ideal. It will allow the joints to work through their normal range, loading the appropriate tissue through the progression from heel strike to push-off.

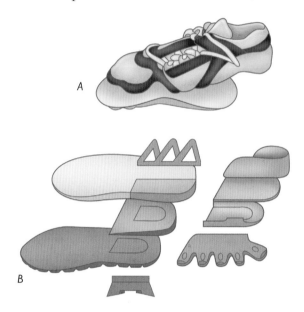

Figure 8.11. The "normal" shoe (A) has many supposedly positive features. Running shoes, in particular, may include "motion control," extra heel cushioning, and a curved longitudinal axis. Some of these features may be necessary for challenged feet, but they will interfere with the natural architecture and function. Thicker soles dampen proprioception; motion control, strangely enough, prevents motion, which also lessens proprioception communication through the body and inhibits some of the normal tissue responses described in this book. The cramped and angled toe box will affect the foot's ability to spread and then push off at an optimal angle. A minimal shoe (B) simply provides protection from the elements and unseen objects. The thin and pliable sole allows the foot to feel the ground and make appropriate responses, while the wide toe box and lack of curving from heel to toe facilitate actions of the metatarsals, from the spreading at heel strike to the correct angle at push-off.

Anything that interferes with joint alignment will affect our ability to use the longer springs of the body. Wearing high heels not only places more weight on the metatarsal heads but also prevents the ankle from dorsiflexing, while cramped or angled toe boxes will force push-off to occur at angles other than the ideal first and second metatarsal heads.

Various "fitness" and "technology" shoes have appeared on the market over the last ten years—many making health and beauty claims. One of the reasons why they claim to "help you lose weight," "burn more calories," or "give you long lean legs" is due to the fact that they alter the body's natural mechanics. We have evolved to make walking as easy and as calorie efficient as possible, so by interfering with that process, we have to compensate with muscle work. When we do so, however, we are also at threat of changing the forces that flow through the joints, making these "technology" shoes unsuitable for many people, if any.

Many people, due to inherited characteristics, accidents, or misuse, no longer have the ideal alignment through the joints of the feet. They may benefit from the use of orthotics to retain efficiency. I believe orthotics to be an intervention of last resort, preferring to use manual therapy, manipulation, and/or exercise to normalize the foot as much as possible. If orthotics are to be used, they should be expertly fitted, and the client should be monitored by an experienced clinician to assess the rest of the body's adaptation to the orthotics. Too often, orthopedic insoles are prescribed, and then the job is considered done. The body will require time, however—and possibly some assistance—to recognize the new position it is in, and so a full screening of the "essential events" should be repeated.

I have two doctors, my left leg and my right.
—G. M. Trevelyan

Walks. The body advances, while the mind flutters around it like a bird.
—Jules Renard

References

Compiled with thanks to Robert Miller.

Arampatzis, Adamantios, Andreas Peper, Stefanie Bierbaum, and Kirsten Albracht. 2010. "Plasticity of Human Achilles Tendon Mechanical and Morphological Properties in Response to Cyclic Strain." *Journal of Biomechanics* 43 (16): 3073–79.

Arampatzis, A., S. Stafilidis, G. DeMonte, K. Karamanidis, G. Morey-Klapsing, and G. P. Brüggemann. 2005. "Strain and Elongation of the Human Gastrocnemius Tendon and Aponeurosis during Maximal Plantarflexion Effort." *Journal of Biomechanics* 38 (4): 833–41.

Ardrey, R. 1961. *African Genesis: A Personal Investigation into the Animal Origins and Nature of Man.* London: Collins.

Beach, P. 2010. *Muscles and Meridians: The Manipulation of Shape.* Edinburgh, UK: Churchill Livingstone Elsevier.

Bell, C. 1837. *The Hand: Its Mechanism and Vital Endowments as Evincing Design.* London: William Pickering.

Biewener, Andrew A. 1998. "Muscle-tendon Stresses and Elastic Energy Storage during Locomotion in the Horse." *Comparative Biochemistry and Physiology: Part B, Biochemistry and Molecular Biology* 120 (1): 73–87.

Blazevich, Anthony. 2011. "The Stretch-Shortening Cycle." In Cardinale, Newton, and Nosaka 2011, 209–22.

Böl, Markus, Heiko Stark, and Nadja Schilling. 2011. "On a Phenomenological Model for Fatigue Effects in Skeletal Muscles." *Journal of Theoretical Biology* 281 (1): 122–32.

Bourke, J. 2011. *What It Means to Be Human: Reflections from 1791 to the Present.* London: Virago.

Bramble, D. M., and D. E. Lieberman. 2004. "Endurance Running and the Evolution of *Homo*." *Nature* 432: 345–52.

Calais-Germain, B. 1993. *Anatomy of Movement.* Seattle, WA: Eastland Press.

Cardinale, M., R. Newton, and K. Nosaka, eds. 2011. *Strength and Conditioning: Biological Principles and Practical Applications.* Oxford: Wiley-Blackwell.

Carmont, M. R., A. M. Highland, J. R. Rochester, E. M. Paling, and M. B. Davies. 2011. "An Anatomical and Radiological Study of the Fascia Cruris and Paratenon of the Achilles Tendon." *Foot and Ankle Surgery* 17 (3): 186–92.

Cochran, Gregory, and Henry Harpending. 2010. *The 10,000 Year Explosion: How Civilization Accelerated Human Evolution.* New York: Basic Books.

Dalton, E., ed. 2011. *Dynamic Body: Exploring Form Expanding Function.* Oklahoma City: Freedom from Pain Institute.

Dalton, E., M. Bishop, M. D. Tillman, and C. J. Hass. 2011. "Simple Change in Standing Position Enhances the Initiation of Gait." *Medicine and Science in Sports and Exercise* 43 (12): 2352–58.

Dart, R. 1996. *Alexander Center.* www.alexandercenter.com/dartspirals.html.

DeRosa, C., and J. A. Porterfield. 2007. "Anatomical Linkages and Muscle Slings of the Lumbopelvic Region." In Vleeming, Mooney, and Stoeckart 2007, 47–62.

Doral, Mahmut Nedim, Mahbub Alam, Murat Bozkurt, Egemen Turhan, Ozgür Ahmet Atay, Gürhan Dönmez, and Nicola Maffulli. 2010. "Functional Anatomy of the Achilles Tendon." *Knee Surgery, Sports Traumatology, Arthroscopy* 18 (5): 638–43.

Earls, James, and Thomas Myers. 2010. *Fascial Release for Structural Balance.* Berkeley, CA: North Atlantic Books.

Filler, A. G. 2007. *The Upright Ape: A New Origin of the Species.* Franklin Lakes, NJ: Career Press.

Franklyn-Miller, A., E. Falvey, R. Clark, A. Bryant, P. Brukner, P. Barker, C. Briggs, P. McCrory. 2009. "The Strain Patterns of the Deep Fascia of the Lower Limb." *Fascia Research II.* Edinburgh, UK: Elsevier.

Fukashiro, Senshi, Dean C. Hay, and Akinori Nagano. 2006. "Biomechanical Behavior of Muscle-Tendon Complex during Dynamic Human Movements." *Journal of Applied Biomechanics* 22 (2): 131–47.

Fukunaga, Tetsuo, Yasuo Kawakami, Keitaro Kubo, and Hiroaki Kanehisa. 2002. "Muscle and Tendon Interaction during Human Movements." *Exercise Sport Science Review* 30 (3): 106–10.

Gracovetsky, S. 2008. *The Spinal Engine.* Montreal: Serge Gracovetsky, PhD.

Hawks, John. 2009. "How Strong Is a Chimpanzee, Really?" *Slate.* February 25. www.slate.com/articles/health_and_science/science/2009/02/how_strong_is_a_chimpanzee.html.

Heinrich, B. 2002. *Why We Run: A Natural History.* New York: Ecco.

Hodges, Paul W., and Kyle Tucker. 2011. "Moving Differently in Pain: A New Theory to Explain the Adaptation to Pain." *Pain* 152: S90–S98.

Huijing, P. A. 1999a. "Muscle as a Collagen Fiber Reinforced Composite Material: Force Transmission in Muscle and Whole Limbs." *Journal of Biomechanics* 32 (4): 329–345.

———. 1999b. "Muscular Force Transmission: A Unified, Dual or Multiple System? A Review and Some Explorative Experimental Results." *Archives of Physiology and Biochemistry* 170 (4): 292–311.

———. 2009. "Epimuscular Myofascial Force Transmission: A Historical Perspective and Implications for New Research." *Journal of Biomechanics* 42: 9–21.

Huijing, P., and G. Baan. 2008. "Myofascial Force Transmission via Extramuscular Pathways Occurs between Antagonistic Muscles." *Cells, Tissues, Organs* 188 (4): 400–414.

Huijing, Peter A., Alper Yaman, Cengizhan Ozturk, and Can A. Yucesoy. 2011. "Effects Angle on Global and Local Strains within Human Triceps Surae Muscle: MRI Analysis Indicating In Vivo Myofascial Force Transmission between Synergistic Muscles." *Surgical and Radiological Anatomy* 33 (10): 869–79.

Ingber, D. 1998. "The Architecture of Life." *Scientific American* 278 (1): 48–57.

Ingold, Tim. 2004. "Culture on the Ground: The World Perceived through the Feet." *Journal of Material Culture* 9 (3): 315–40.

Inwood, S. 2003. *The Forgotten Genius: The Biography of Robert Hooke, 1635–1703.* San Francisco: MacAdam/Cage.

Ireland, Mary Lloyd, John D. Willson, Bryon T. Ballantyne, and Irene McClay Davis. 2003. "Hip Strength in Females with and without Patellofemoral Pain." *Journal of Orthopaedic and Sports Physical Therapy* 33 (11): 671–76.

Jaspers, R. T., R. Brunner, U. N. Riede, and P. A. Huijing. 2005. "Healing of the Aponeurosis during Recovery from Aponeurotomy: Morphological and Histological Adaptation and Related Changes in Mechanical Properties." *Journal of Orthopaedic Research* 23 (2): 266–73.

Jielile, Jiasharete, Jing Ping Bai, Gulnur Sabirhazi, Darebai Redat, Tuoheti Yilihamu, Baoltri Xinlin, Geyang Hu, Bin Tang, Bing Liang, and Qi Sun. 2010. "Factors Influencing the Tensile Strength of Repaired Achilles Tendon: A Biomechanical Experiment Study." *Clinical Biomechanics* 25 (8): 789–95.

Kawakami, Y., T. Muraoka, S. Ito, H. Kanehisa, and T. Fukunaga. 2002. "In Vivo Muscle Fibre Behaviour during Counter-movement Exercise in Humans Reveals a Significant Role for Tendon Elasticity." *Journal of Physiology* 540 (2): 635–46.

Kendall, F. P., E. K. McCreary, P. G. Provance, M. M. Rodgers, and W. A. Romani. 2005. *Muscles: Testing and Function with Posture and Pain.* Baltimore, MD: Lippincott, Williams and Wilkins.

Kjaer, M. 2004. "Role of Extracellular Matrix in Adaptation of Tendon and Skeletal Muscle to Mechanical Loading." *Physiological Reviews* 84 (2): 649–98.

Kjaer, M., H. Langberg, K. Heinemeier, M. L. Bayer, M. Hansen, L. Holm, S. Doessing, M. Kongsgaard, M. R. Krogsgaard, and S. P. Magnusson. 2009. "From Mechanical Loading to Collagen Synthesis, Structural Changes and Function in Human Tendon." *Scandinavian Journal of Medicine and Science in Sports* 19 (4): 500–510.

Komi, P., ed. 2011. *Neuromuscular Aspects of Sport Performance*. Chichester, UK: Blackwell.

Kongsgaard, M., C. H. Nielson, S. Hegnsvad, P. Aagaard, and S. P. Magnusson. 2011. "Mechanical Properties of the Human Achilles Tendon, In Vivo." *Clinical Biomechanics* 26 (7): 772–77.

Latash, M. L. 2012. *Fundamentals of Motor Control*. Waltham, MA: Academic Press.

Levin, S. M. 2007. "A Suspensory System for the Sacrum in Pelvic Mechanics: Biotensegrity." In Vleeming, Mooney, and Stoeckart 2007, 229–38.

Lichtwark, G. A., and A. M. Wilson. 2007. "Is Achilles Tendon Compliance Optimised for Maximum Muscle Efficiency during Locomotion?" *Journal of Biomechanics* 40 (8): 1768–75.

Lieberman, D. E. 2011. *The Evolution of the Human Head*. Cambridge, MA: Belknap Press of Harvard University Press.

Lovejoy, C. O. 2007. "Evolution of the Human Lumbopelvic Region and Its Relationship to Some Clinical Deficits of the Spine and Pelvis." In Vleeming, Mooney, and Stoeckart 2007, 141–58.

Maloiy, M. O. et al. 1986. "Energetic Cost of Carrying Loads: Have African Women Discovered an Economic Way?" *Nature* 319: 668–69.

Malvankar, S., and Khan, W. S. 2011. "Evolution of the Achilles Tendon: The Athlete's Achilles Heel?" *Foot* 21 (4): 193–97.

Maus, H. M., S. W. Lipfert, M. Gross, J. Rummel, and A. Seyfarth. 2010. "Upright Human Gait Did Not Provide a Major Mechanical Challenge for Our Ancestors." *Nature Communications* September 7.

McArdle, W. D. 2010. *Exercise Physiology: Nutrition, Energy and Human Performance*. New York: Lippincott, Williams and Wilkins.

McCredie, S. 2007. *Balance: In Search of the Lost Sense*. New York: Little, Brown.

McDougall, C. 2010. *Born to Run: The Hidden Tribe, the Ultra-runners and the Greatest Race the World Has Never Seen*. London: Profile Books.

McNeill Alexander, R. 1986. "Human Energetics: Making Headway in Africa." *Nature* 319: 623–24.

—. 1992. *The Human Machine: How the Body Works*. London: Natural History Museum.

—. 1995. "Elasticity in Mammalian Backs." Second Interdisciplinary World Conference on Low Back Pain: The Integrated Function of the Lumbar Spine and Sacroiliac Joints.

—. 2002. "Tendon Elasticity and Muscle Function." *Comparative Biochemistry and Physiology: Part A, Molecular and Integrative Physiology* 133 (4): 1001–11.

—. 2005. *Energy for Animal Life*. Oxford: Oxford University Press.

—. 2006. *Principles of Animal Locomotion*. Princeton, NJ: Princeton University Press.

Meredith, M. 2011. *Born in Africa: The Quest for the Origins of Human Life*. London: Simon and Schuster.

Michaud, T. 2011. *Human Locomotion: The Conservative Management of Gait-Related Disorders*. Newton, MA: Newton Biomechanics.

Middleditch, A., and J. Oliver. 2005. *Functional Anatomy of the Spine*. Edinburgh, UK: Elsevier.

Morgan, E. 1990. *The Scars of Evolution: What Our Bodies Tell Us about Human Origins*. Worcester, UK: Billing and Sons.

Morton, D. J. 1952. *Human Locomotion and Body Form: A Study of Gravity and Man*. Baltimore, MD: Williams and Wilkins.

Muller, D., and R. Schleip. 2011. "Fascial Fitness: Fascia Oriented Training for Bodywork and Movement Therapies." *Terra Rosa* 7: 2–11. www.terrarosa.com.au/articles/Terra_News7.pdf.

Muscolino, J. 2006. *Kinesiology: The Skeletal System and Muscle Function*. St. Louis, MO: Mosby.

Myers, T. W. 2009. *Anatomy Trains: Myofascial Meridians for Manual and Movement Therapists*. Edinburgh, UK: Churchill Livingstone Elsevier.

Nicholson, G. 2009. *The Lost Art of Walking: The History, Science, Philosophy, and Literature of Pedestrianism*. New York: Riverhead Books.

O'Keefe, James H., Robert Vogel, Carl J. Lavie, and Loren Cordain. 2011. "Exercise Like a Hunter-Gatherer: A Prescription for Organic Physical Fitness." *Progress in Cardiovascular Diseases* 53 (6): 471–79.

Olsen, B. D. 2009. *Understanding Human Anatomy through Evolution*. Morrisville, NC: Lulu Press.

Ortega, J. D., and C. T. Farley. 2005. "Minimizing Center of Mass Vertical Movement Increases Metabolic Cost in Walking." *Journal of Applied Physiology* 99 (6): 2099–107.

Oschman, J. 2003. *Energy Medicine in Therapeutics and Human Performance*. Edinburgh, UK: Butterworth Heinemann.

Parker, P. J., and C. A. Briggs. 2007. "Anatomy and Biomechanics of the Lumbar Fasciae: Implications for Lumbopelvic Control and Clinical Practice." In Vleeming, Mooney, and Stoeckart 2007, 63–74.

Perry, J., and J. M. Burnfield. 2010. *Gait Analysis*. Thorofare, NJ: Slack.

Pichler, W., N. P. Tesch, W. Grechenig, O. Leithgoeb, and G. Windisch. 2007. "Anatomic Variations of the Musculotendinous Junction of the Soleus Muscle and Its Clinical Implications." *Clinical Anatomy* 20 (4): 444–47.

Pontzer, H., J. H. Holloway, D. A. Raichlen, and D. E. Lieberman. 2009. "Control and Function of Arm Swing in Human Walking and Running." *Journal of Experimental Biology* 212 (6): 894.

Powers, Christopher M. n.d. *Biomechanical Factors Contributing to Patellofemoral Pain; The Dynamic QAngle*. Musculoskeletal Biomechanics Research Lab, University of Southern California.

———. n.d. *Dynamic Stabilization of the Patellofemoral Joint: Stabilization from Above and Below*. Musculoskeletal Biomechanics Research Lab, University of Southern California.

———. 2003. "The Influence of Altered Lower-Extremity Kinematics on Patellofemoral Joint Dysfunction: A Theoretical Perspective." *Journal of Orthopaedic and Sports Physical Therapy* 33 (11): 639–46.

———. 2010. "The Influence of Abnormal Hip Mechanics on Knee Injury: A Biomechanical Perspective." *Journal of Orthopaedic and Sports Physical Therapy* 40 (2): 42–51.

Powers, Christopher M., Samuel R. Ward, Michael Fredericson, Marc Guillet, and Frank G. Shellock. 2003. "Patellofemoral Kinematics during Weight-bearing and Non-weight-bearing Knee Extension in Persons with Lateral Subluxation of the Patella: A Preliminary Study." *Journal of Orthopaedic and Sports Physical Therapy* 33 (11): 677–85.

Premkumar, K. 2004. *The Massage Connection: Anatomy and Physiology*. Baltimore, MD: Lippincott, Williams and Wilkins.

Richards, J. 2008. *Biomechanics in Clinic and Research*. Edinburgh, UK: Churchill Livingstone Elsevier.

Sahrmann, S. A. 2002. *Diagnosis and Treatment of Movement Impairment Syndromes*. St. Louis, MO: Mosby.

Sawicki, Gregory S., Cara L. Lewis, and Daniel P. Ferris. 2009. "It Pays to Have a Spring in Your Step." *Exercise and Sport Sciences Reviews* 37 (3): 130–38.

Saxby, L. 2011. *Proprioception: Making Sense of Barefoot Running*. London: Terra Plana International.

Schleip, R., T. W. Findley, L. Chaitow, and P. Huijing. 2012. *Fascia: The Tensional Network of the Human Body*. Edinburgh, UK: Churchill Livingstone Elsevier.

Shubin, N. 2008. *Your Inner Fish: A Journey into the 3.5-billion-year History of the Human Body*. London: Allen Lane.

Solnit, R. 2002. *Wanderlust: A History of Walking*. London: Verso.

Stringer, C. 2011. *The Origin of Our Species*. London: Allen Lane.

Stringer, C., and P. Andrews. 2011. *The Complete World of Human Evolution*. London: Thames and Hudson.

Tattersall, I. 2007. *Becoming Human: Evolution and Human Uniqueness*. Oxford: Oxford University Press.

Tudge, C., and J. Young. 2009. *The Link: Uncovering Our Earliest Ancestors.* London: Little, Brown.

Verkhoshansky, Y., and M. Siff. 2009. *Supertraining.* Rome: Ultimate Athletic Concepts.

Vleeming, A., V. Mooney, and R. Stoeckart, eds. 2007. *Movement, Stability and Lumbopelvic Pain: Integration of Research and Therapy.* Edinburgh, UK: Elsevier.

Vleeming A., R. Stoeckart, A. C. W. Volkers, and C. J. Snijders. 1990. "Relation between Form and Function in the Sacroiliac Joint. Part 1: Clinical Anatomical Concepts." *Spine* 15 (2): 130–32.

Vleeming A., A. C. W. Volkers, C. J. Snijders, and R. Stoeckart. 1990. "Relation between Form and Function in the Sacroiliac Joint. Part 2: Biomechanical Aspects." *Spine* 15 (2): 133–36.

Vogel, S. 2001. *Prime Mover: A Natural History of Muscle.* New York: W. W. Norton.

White, Tim D., and Pieter A. Folkens. 2005. *The Human Bone Manual.* Edinburgh, UK: Elsevier.

Wrangham, R. 2009. *Catching Fire: How Cooking Made Us Human.* London: Profile Books.

Wynn, T., and F. L. Coolidge. 2012. *How to Think Like a Neandertal.* New York: Oxford University Press.

Yahia, L. H., P. Pigeon, and E. A. DesRosiers. 1993. "Viscoelastic Properties of the Human Lumbodorsal Fascia." *Journal of Biomedical Engineering* 15 (5): 425–29.

Zorn, A. 2007a. "Physical Forms about Structure: The Elasticity of Fascia." *Structural Integration* (March): 15–17.

—. 2007b. "The Swingwalkers of Zambia." *Structural Integration* (December): 20–21.

Zorn, A., and K. Hodeck. 2011. "Walk with Elastic Fascia: Use the Springs in Your Step!" In Dalton 2011, 96–123.

Index

Waiter's tray. *see* Sustentaculum talus
Walking, 14. *see also* Spiral line; Triangulation;
    aspect of human motion, 14; bipedal gait, 49;
    communication of force, 16; controlled falling,
    13; elements of, 15; in evolution, 21; factors
    in, 14; impact of foot on ground, 15; gait
    cycle divisions, 52; gravity and, 17; ground
    reaction force, 18–21; lateral stability, 49; line of
    support, 48, 49; lower limb mechanics, 125–127;
    lumbar-extension, 23; movement strategies, 22;
    myofascial tissues response, 15; proprioceptors,
    15, 16; propulsion, 47; shock absorption, 47,
    50–51; for stability, 191; stages of gait, 52;
    stance stability, 47, 48; system coordination in,
    13; theories on, 14; thoracolumbar fascia in,
    34; and time dimension, 16–17; whole body
    involvement, 14–15
Weight acceptance, 62–65
Wider toe box, 200
Windlass effect, 80. *see also* Catapult mechanism;
    Achilles tendon on, 81; exercise on, 82; factors
    in, 83

Z stretch, 160; and hip position, 174

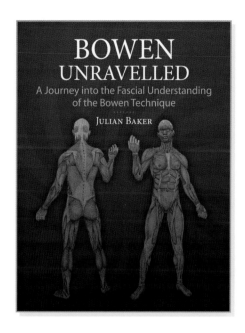

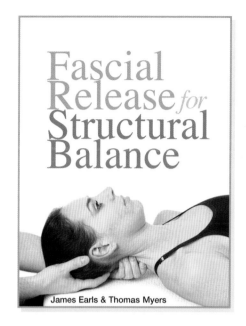

BOWEN UNRAVELLED: A JOURNEY INTO THE FASCIAL UNDERSTANDING OF THE BOWEN TECHNIQUE

Julian Baker • 978 1 905367 40 5 (UK) 978 1 583947 65 4 (US) • £16.99 / $29.95 • 168 pages • 275 x 212mm • paperback

The Bowen Technique, named after its originator Tom Bowen, has grown hugely in popularity since it was first taught in the 1980s. This book breaks down the concepts of The Bowen Technique and develops an understanding of what is going on during a treatment, including explanations of why things happen the way that they do.

Julian Baker is the principal of the European College of Bowen Studies, and is one of the world's leading experts on The Bowen Technique, fascia and connective tissue.

FASCIAL RELEASE FOR STRUCTURAL BALANCE

James Earls and Thomas Myers • 978 1 905367 18 4 (UK) 978 1 556439 37 7 (US) • £24.99 / $34.95 • 288 pages • 275 x 212mm • paperback

Fascial Release for Structural Balance combines manual therapy skills with the exciting new field of structural therapy, which employs the unique and newly discovered properties of fascial tissues. Through informed assessment and manipulation of fascial patterns, you can help eradicate many of your clients' chronic strain patterns—for good.

The book is designed for any bodywork practitioner using manual therapy who can help their current and future clients by giving them a structural analysis and creating a treatment strategy using the techniques included in this book. The authors bring together a unique introduction to fascially informed structural anatomy with a method for postural analysis and detailed and easily applied techniques.

Thomas Myers has practiced integrative structural therapy for over 30 years in a variety of clinical and cultural settings. He is the author of *Anatomy Trains* (Elsevier 2001, 2009) and numerous collected articles for journals and trade publications.

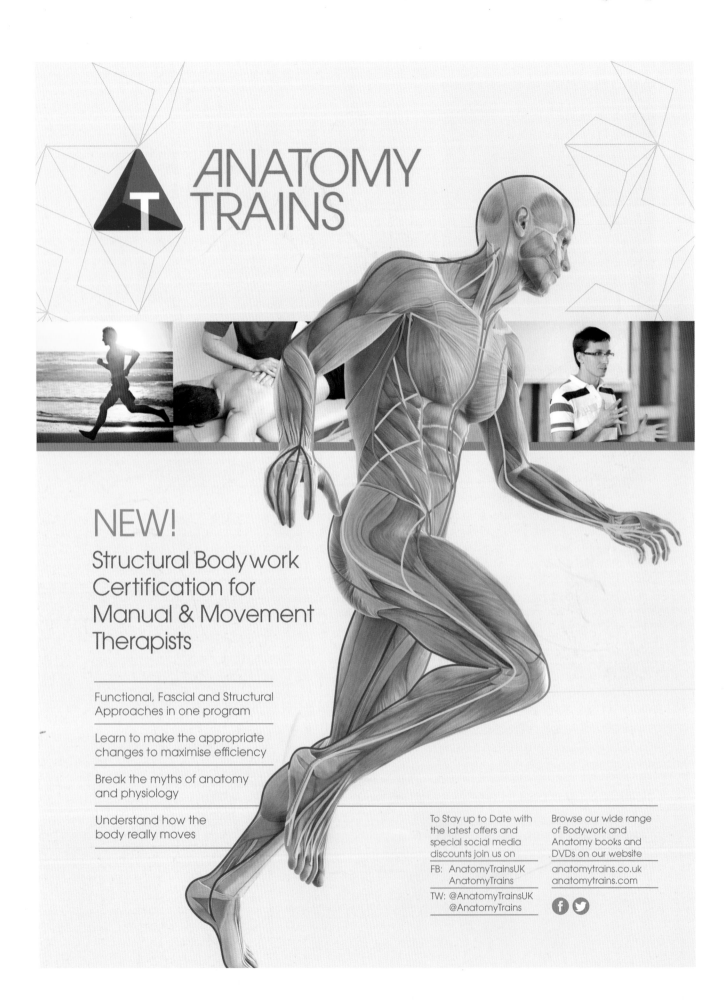